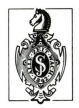

Tim Chard · Arnold Klopper

Placental Function Tests

With 23 Figures

Springer-Verlag
Berlin Heidelberg New York 1982

Michael R. K. Pruggmayer
Dipl.-Biol., Arzt

Tim Chard, MD, FRCOG
Professor of Obstetrics, Gynaecology
and Reproductive Physiology
St Bartholomew's Hospital Medical College
and the London Hospital Medical College
London, UK.

Arnold Klopper, MD, FRCOG
Professor of Reproductive Endocrinology
Department of Obstetrics and Gynaecology
Royal Infirmary, Foresterhill
Aberdeen, UK.

ISBN 3-540-11529-3 Springer-Verlag Berlin Heidelberg New York
ISBN 0-387-11529-3 Springer-Verlag New York Heidelberg Berlin

Library of Congress Cataloging in Publication Data
Chard, T. Placental function tests. Bibliography: p. Includes index. 1. Placental function tests. 2. Placenta — diseases — Diagnosis. I. Klopper, Arnold. II. Title. [DNLM: 1. Placental function tests. WQ 212 C741p] RG591.C47   618.3'4   82-5709
ISBN 0-387-11529-3 (U.S.) AACR2

This work is subject to copyright. All rights are reserved, whether the whole or part of the material is concerned, specifically those of translation, reprinting, re-use of illustrations, broadcasting, reproduction by photocopying machine or similar means, and storage in data banks. Under §54 of the German Copyright Law where copies are made for other than private use, a fee is payable to 'Verwertungsgesellschaft Wort', Munich.

© by Springer-Verlag Berlin Heidelberg 1982
Printed in Great Britain

The use of registered names, trademarks, etc. in this publication does not imply, even in the absence of a specific statement, that such names are exempt from the relevant protective laws and regulations and therefore free for general use.

Filmset by Photo-Graphics, Stockland, Nr. Honiton, Devon
Printed and bound by Spottiswoode Ballantyne Ltd, Colchester, Essex

2128/3916-543210

Preface

Biochemical tests of fetal well-being ('placental function tests') have been part of routine obstetric practice for more than twenty years. This book provides an overview of the current status of these tests — the physiological basis for their use, and their advantages and limitations in clinical practice. Considerable attention is given to interpretation, a subject which in the past has led to much confusion both in the scientific literature and in the minds of clinicians. Recent advances are described in detail, in particular the discovery of a whole new generation of placental products some of which offer great promise in the prediction of conditions, such as placental abruption and premature labour, which cannot be identified by any other current parameters. Finally, a set of clear recommendations is put forward for the choice of test in most of the common complications of both early and late pregnancy. The emphasis throughout is on how the basic biology of fetoplacental products dictates their use and interpretation in pathological conditions.

London and Aberdeen,   Tim Chard
March 1982.   Arnold Klopper

Contents

Chapter 1. Introduction 1

Chapter 2. The Biology and Measurement of Fetoplacental Products 4

   Specific biochemical products of the human fetoplacental unit 4
   Site of synthesis of placental products 5
   Trophoblast products 7
   Trophoblast products in relation to obstetric pathology 14
   References 16

Chapter 3. Analysis of the Clinical Results of Placental Function Tests 18

   Definition of normality 18
   Definition of abnormality 20
   Numerical definition of normal range 23
   How useful is a test? Analysis of clinical efficiency ... 26
   Other aspects of the analysis of placental function tests 28
   References 33

Chapter 4. Placental Enzymes 34

   Chemistry, synthesis and metabolism 34
   Functions 35
   Measurement 35
   Maternal levels in normal pregnancy 35
   Clinical application of HSAP and CAP measurement in maternal serum 35
   Other placental enzymes of potential clinical interest ... 36
   References 38

Chapter 5. Steroid Hormones 39

   Oestrogens 39
   Oestriol 40

Other oestrogens	53
Progestogens	53
References	54

Chapter 6. Placental Protein Hormones (hCG and hPL) — 56

Discovery	56
Chemistry	56
Synthesis	57
Metabolism	57
Biological functions	58
Control mechanisms	58
Measurement	59
Time-to-time variation	60
Normal range	60
Clinical applications of measurement	60
Conclusions — hPL levels in the management of late pregnancy	67
References	68

Chapter 7. Other Placental Proteins — 70

Discovery of new placental proteins	70
Schwangerschaftsprotein 1 (SP1)	71
Clinical applications of SP1 measurement	73
Placental protein 5 (PP5)	76
Clinical applications of PP5 measurement	76
Pregnancy-associated plasma protein A (PAPP-A)	78
References	80

Chapter 8. Conclusions: Choice and Use of Placental Function Tests — 83

Placental function tests in antenatal care — are they worthwhile?	83
Interpretation of placental function tests	86
Placental function tests as screening tests	90
Choice of test	90
References	92

Subject Index 93

Chapter 1
Introduction

Antenatal care in this century has undergone a sea change. It began as a charitable concern for the indigent, often unmarried, mother. As, one by one, the causes of maternal death were eliminated, the focus of care shifted to her unborn baby. Now we are approaching the point where nearly every established pregnancy ends in the birth of a live, surviving baby, and the proper concern of antenatal care is with the quality of the product. This book is written at the transition point. Obstetricians can make reasonably reliable guesses as to whether a fetus has a better chance of survival in the uterus or out of it; obstetric services can produce it alive and paediatricians can keep it alive. But there our powers end. We can do very little about the loss of life before pregnancy is established and no more about treating the ills which might beset the fetus in utero. Our purpose is to examine some of the means which might be used to determine how far the fetus is affected by the hazards of pregnancy and thus to provide some forecast of the outcome. With perinatal deaths ranging from 12 to 20 per 1000 births in Britain, we still have some way to go before every baby which can be saved, survives. It is here that biochemical monitoring of the fetus can make a contribution to the choice of the few alternative lines of action open to us.

Present-day antenatal care consists largely of diagnosis. Three means are available for determining whether there is an increased risk to the life or health of the fetus. The first lies in the clinical facts of the situation—the mother's age, parity, nutrition, social class or past obstetric history and maternal disease such as pre-eclampsia, diabetes or erythroblastosis. The second is instrumental examination of the fetus—ultrasound measurements, cardiotocography, fetoscopy, amniocentesis. The third is the measurement of fetoplacental products in maternal body fluids. Although from time to time comparisons with the first two means of fetal risk assessment will have to be made, this book is entirely concerned with the third: biochemical measurement of placental function in the broad sense.

Fetal diagnosis presents two major problems. This first is the inaccessibility of the fetus and the second is the difficulty of describing the precise condition of the child even when it is delivered. There are very few measurements which can be made on the delivered baby which have any relevance either to its state of health or future development to set against the figure provided by the antepartum biochemical measurement of placental function. The fetus is either alive or dead. The Apgar score generally reflects what happened in the last few hours before birth, a long time after the placental function measurement was made. The baby can be weighed, a useful enough procedure for studies of fetal growth, but not relevant to many other aspects of fetal wellbeing. Only 15 in every 1000 babies die and often enough with conditions like anencephaly, it does not require placental function tests to determine the outcome in advance. In the absence of reliable figures for the fetal state to set against the figures of biochemical measurements the clinician is freed of any constraints in deciding how accurately the placental function test predicted the fetal state. Not surprisingly, beliefs about the value of a particular placental function test often say more about the clinician operating the test than about the value of the test.

In this situation our first endeavour will be to consider what objective means there are to examine the value of any test of placental function. To this end one might choose a number of findings which have a relationship to neonatal health and search out how far any particular placental function test is able to predict such findings. An illustrative, but by no means comprehensive, list of such findings is given in Table 1.1. We propose to examine the common placental function tests with respect to Table 1.1. We do not propose to enter the field of methodology, but merely, given an adequate method of measurement, to consider how best the results of that measurement can be made to reflect any or all of the ills in Table 1.1.

Table 1.1. Aspects of fetal state which might be predicted by placental function tests[a]

1	Perinatal death, stillbirth or neonatal death
2	Intrauterine growth retardation
3	Fetal distress in labour
4	Neonatal asphyxia
5	Postnatal motor and intellectual impairment
6	Premature delivery
7	Congenital abnormalities
8	Specific diseases, such as erythroblastosis, metabolic and nutritional disorders induced by maternal diabetes

[a] The term 'placental function tests' is used because of its familiarity rather than its accuracy. Thus, the prime use of these tests is to determine 'fetal function', and in some instances they measure fetal as well as placental products.

Table 1.2. Obstetric management which might be influenced by placental function tests

1	Pre-term delivery, either caesarean section or induction of labour
2	Bedrest
3	Observation, including fetal monitoring in labour
4	Drugs, e.g. hypotensives or β mimetics
5	Operative intervention in labour
6	Neonatal intensive care
7	Termination of pregnancy for congenital abnormality

Although treatment is not the prime objective of a placental function test, the results do have a bearing on treatment. Table 1.2 lists some of the lines of treatment which might be affected when placental function tests have helped to locate an at-risk pregnancy. Many factors enter into the decision, say, between immediate induction of labour or further bed rest. Placental function tests should not be definitive in such a choice. They are most appropriately used in conjunction with all the clinical findings. A fall in urinary oestriol output in a young multipara at 38 weeks with a mild pre-eclampsia does not mean much. The same fall in an elderly primigravida just past term could well tip the balance in favour of caesarean section. We will try to define the true value and use of placental function tests in obstetric practice.

Chapter 2
The Biology and Measurement of Fetoplacental Products

The concept upon which placental function tests is based, is superficially simple. The conceptus secretes a unique product into the mother. Measurement of this product or its metabolites in the mother's blood or urine reflects the secretion rate of the product and hence the overall function of the placenta or the wellbeing of the fetus. High levels indicate that function is good; low levels show that it is unsatisfactory. This is an oversimplification which has given rise to many difficulties in clinical practice and led to much disenchantment about the usefulness of biochemical tests of placental function. The difficulty arises because it is not possible to draw a sharp line between normal and abnormal; at best there is a wide 'grey' area between the two and, upon occasion, measurements well into the abnormal zone are associated with an entirely normal outcome, and vice versa.

The evaluation of a placental function test rests upon the analysis of this 'grey' area; it is central to our purpose and will be pursued in Chapter 3. Here we will consider in what manner fetoplacental biology, such as the synthesis and metabolism of placental products, may influence the results of placental function tests. Often pathological states, such as those detailed in Table 1.1, have little influence on the synthesis of placental products, and can be of no use in determining the types of management outlined in Table 1.2. It is essential to the intelligent use of placental function tests to have a good grasp of the biology of placental products and how they may be affected by particular pathological processes such as retarded fetal growth.

Specific biochemical products of the human fetoplacental unit

At first sight the definition of a specific product of the fetoplacental unit seems simple: it is something which only the placenta, or the fetus and placenta acting in concert, can produce. It is therefore not present in males or non-pregnant females. In the case of the steroids, however, this distinction is obviously merely quantitative. The ovary, the testis and the adrenal can, and do, produce the full range of steroids which the fetoplacental unit can synthesize. The difference is merely one of scale. A pregnant woman at term excretes perhaps ten thousand times as much oestriol in the urine as a male does. Even then it is a matter of which steroid you choose; the plasma concentration of progesterone in pregnancy seldom exceeds ten times the concentration in the non-pregnant luteal phase. As techniques for the measurement of 'specific' placental polypeptides have become more and more sensitive it has become clear that they too, are by no means unique to pregnancy. Trace quantities of most of these placental proteins have been detected in individuals who were not carrying any placental tissue. It is accepted that the ability to synthesize these proteins is not limited to the trophoblast. Other cells may carry the code in a genetically repressed state. Occasionally adult cells, notably tumour cells or fibroblasts, become de-repressed and synthesize and secrete 'specific' placental proteins. In practice the difference between trophoblastic production and that of other tissues is so large that it does not give rise to any difficulty in the interpretation of placental function tests. The small potential contribution of non-trophoblastic tissues is only of significance in tests for the detection of pregnancy.

Site of synthesis of placental products

In the human the maternal and fetal blood streams are separated by at least two layers of cells: the vascular endothelium of the fetal capillaries, and the trophoblast. The latter comprises two types of cell: syncytiotrophoblast, which is a continuous layer on the surface of the villi; and cytotrophoblast, consisting of isolated cells which are abundant in the early placenta but become very sparse towards term. Internal to the trophoblast is a basement membrane which may play an important role in the barrier function of the placenta (Panigel 1974). On the outer surface of the syncytiotrophoblast, adjacent to the maternal intervillous space, is a 'turf' of microvilli (Ludwig 1974); these effectively enhance the total area available for exchange between mother and fetus, estimated by previous workers to be 11 m^2. These microvilli are assuming a place of some importance in placental physiology. They greatly enlarge the secreting surface of the placenta and constitute the ultimate point of entry of placental products into the maternal circulation. By breaking off they may be a means of entry of placental products other than by active secretion.

Although some biosynthetic activity goes on in the stroma and possibly in the walls of the fetal blood vessels, the syncytiotrophoblast is by far and away the main source of the placental proteins. In some respects acceptance of the syncytiotrophoblast as the sole and exclusive site for the synthesis of pregnancy-associated products has been too facile. Diczfalusy (1962), in developing the concept of the fetoplacental unit, was the first to find flaws in this article of faith. Even in this case, critical steps in the formation of steroid hormones from fetal precursors take place in the syncytiotrophoblast; which is why the clinical interpretation of oestrogen values is very similar to that of the exclusively placental products.

From time to time, doubts are raised as to whether the trophoblast is the sole source of the polypeptides associated with the placenta (Gau and Chard 1976; Klopper et al. 1979). Although it is beyond question that the trophoblast is the pre-eminent site for the synthesis of the products considered in this book, the experimental basis on which this belief rests is often shaky. In many cases it consists of little more than the demonstration of a particular protein in the syncytiotrophoblast. The same tissue also has binders for a number of maternal proteins, e.g. ferritin, and is permeable to others like immunoglobulins. Furthermore the tendency to allocate products characteristic of pregnancy to the trophoblast has helped to obscure the biosynthetic activity of a closely opposed tissue, that of the decidua. This has been shown to be a source of prolactin in pregnancy. It may also be the site of synthesis of pregnancy-associated plasma protein A.

Ultramicroscopic studies suggest that there is functional subspecialisation within the syncytiotrophoblast: this tissue appears to be divided into thin areas which overlie fetal capillaries and are obviously specialised for transport, and thicker areas, not adjacent to fetal capillaries, which contain those structures (ribosomes, endoplasmic reticulum) usually associated with synthesis (Burgos and Rodrigues 1966) (Fig. 2.1). Implicit in these observations is the possibility that measurement of a synthetic function might not reflect the transfer functions (nutrients, blood gases, waste products) which are obviously all-important in the study of fetal wellbeing. However, there is little or no evidence that these aspects of trophoblast activity can vary independently of each other. For all practical purposes it is assumed that the trophoblast functions as a whole, and that a decline in one activity reflects a decline in all activities.

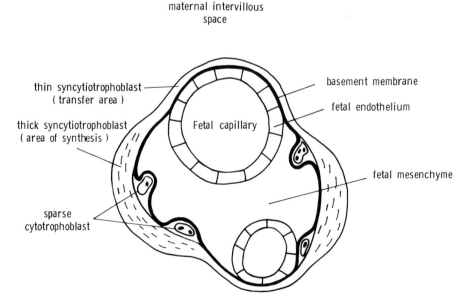

Fig. 2.1. Diagram of a chorionic villus surrounded by the maternal intervillous space. Note the thick areas which contain the organelles for synthetic functions and the thin areas overlying fetal capillaries (vasculo-syncytial membranes) which are presumably specialised for transfer.

Trophoblast products

Mechanism of synthesis

There is no reason to believe that synthetic mechanisms in the trophoblast are different from comparable mechanisms in other tissues. Thus the production of steroids depends on a sequence of enzyme activities in the cytosol and mitochondria; the production of proteins on the translation of messenger RNA (mRNA) by ribosomes. Similarly, the detailed mechanism for the export of these products across the cell membrane is unlikely to differ from other tissues (a process which is anyway poorly understood).

There is, however, one feature which is quite unique to the trophoblast. This is that the cell membrane abuts directly on to the bloodstream in the intervillous space (Fig. 2.1), whereas all other secretory cells in the body are separated from the bloodstream by, at least, a layer of blood vessel endothelium and its basement membrane.[1] It may be that this anatomical relationship is the key to the understanding of the rather remarkable biology of the human trophoblast.

This anatomical relationship has some bearing on the fact that the placental proteins are secreted almost exclusively into the maternal circulation. On the maternal face of the trophoblast there is free access of the trophoblast products to the maternal circulation. On the other side there are barriers between the trophoblast and the fetal circulation. Perhaps the most formidable of these is the basement membrane of the trophoblast but others include the mesenchymal stroma of the chorionic villi and the basement membrane and endothelium of the fetal capillaries. The levels of placental proteins are invariably one or more orders of magnitude higher in the maternal than in the fetal circulation and, when the relative volumes of the two circulations are taken into account, it is likely that the presence of placental proteins in the fetus is the result of leakage without any functional significance. The same reasoning does not apply to the steroid hormones. They pass back and forth from fetal to maternal circulation. The concentration of oestriol and progesterone is higher in the fetus than in the mother and there is no equilibrium between the two compartments. On such grounds these are as likely to be fetal as maternal hormones.

Distribution

The distribution of placental proteins in various fetal compartments once they leave the placenta has no practical significance. The concentration of steroids in various fetal compartments may be more meaningful, particularly if they have any fetal function. The inaccessibility of the fetal compartments, however, puts such measurements beyond the realms of practicability. The one

---

[1] A possible exception to this argument is the whole group of neurotransmitter substances: molecules released at a nerve ending which act across a synapse without traversing other cells.

exception is amniotic fluid. It has been argued that, with respect to oestriol concentration, amniotic fluid could be regarded as an extracorporeal part of the fetal circulation (Klopper 1972). This somewhat fanciful notion never made much headway; partly because the concentration of oestriol in amniotic fluid did not bear a notably close relationship to the fetal state and partly because amniocentesis, particularly repeated amniocentesis, is not practical in the context of placental function tests. The distribution of placental products in the fetal compartments and their putative function there, remains unknown territory.

In the mother, the models for the distribution of placental proteins and for steroids is quite different, and from the point of view of placental function tests, much in favour of the former. Proteins, being big molecules, make their way out of the intravascular compartment with difficulty and to a small extent. They do not penetrate beyond the interstitial fluid and their plasma concentration is largely an outcome of the balance between three variables—plasma volume, metabolic removal and the rate of input from the placenta. The situation with the steroids is different. A large proportion of the total steroid in the mother's body is held in the interstitial fluid and some within the cells. More steroid is held in body fat and to complicate matters further, a good deal of the placental production of, say oestriol, passes into the enterohepatic circulation and is locked away from the other compartments for varying periods. Thus the concentration of a steroid in the maternal plasma is the outcome, not simply of inflow from the placenta, but of movements between compartments and of criss-crossing metabolic pathways.

Metabolism

The distribution and eventual breakdown or excretion of the fetoplacental steroid hormones in the mother is a complex process. Knowledge of the metabolic products of the steroids in blood and urine is also important to the understanding of the clinical use of a test. With the trophoblast proteins, by contrast, a simple generalisation is possible: they are all metabolised principally in the kidneys and liver, and a small proportion (around 1%) is excreted in the urine. Any more detailed knowledge than this is irrelevant to clinical application.

Two aspects of the metabolism of placental products are relevant to their measurement. These are the half-life and the time-to-time variation. Half-life is important because, apparently, the shorter the half-life of a product the more rapidly will its levels reflect a decrease in fetoplacental function. If this were the sole criterion it would give a major advantage to a material such as placental lactogen (hPL), with a half-life of about 15 min, or the steroids, which have even shorter half-lives. Yet this advantage is not realised in practice. The reason is that most situations in which placental function tests are of value are long standing rather than acute. The time-scale of fetal growth retardation is measured in weeks rather than hours, and under these circumstances half-life is unimportant. Acute events in the antepartum period, like premature labour or antepartum haemorrhage, do not cast a shadow before them. They are difficult to predict by any parameter. Biochemical changes after an acute event are of limited value in clinical management.

Time-to-time variation is composed of several elements. The first originates in methodology. At the present time most measurements of placental products are done by radioimmunoassay (RIA). Under the best circumstances the coefficient of variation of replicate measurements in a single run (intra-assay precision) is 8%–10%. (The coefficient of variation is the standard deviation of replicates expressed as a percentage of the mean.) The inter-assay precision, which applies when serial measurements of a placental product are made, runs at 10%–12%. Not surprisingly it is difficult to detect other forms of time-to-time variation above this technical noise level and claims to have demonstrated biological rhythms in the production of placental products have not been convincing. This applies particularly to the measurement of placental proteins. Although claims that the plasma concentration of some placental proteins may follow a set pattern of peak and nadir within the 24 hours have been published, more detailed studies in which the data have been analysed in depth have failed to show a pattern. In the case of steroids, like oestriol, the evidence for a diurnal variation, although not strong, is better than for the proteins. There is at least a reasonable theoretical basis for such a rhythm. Adrenal steroid production shows a clear diurnal rhythm. Substrate supply is a likely limiting factor in placental oestrogen production, and if a substantial proportion of the substrate for oestrogen biosynthesis is derived from the maternal adrenals, this is likely to show fluctuation in keeping with her adrenal rhythms. In practice the largely theoretical problems of diurnal rhythms are easily overcome by taking samples at a fixed time of day.

The factors involved in the urinary excretion of placental products vary from those concerned in the variation of plasma concentration. Proteins are seldom measured in urine and the variability of their excretion is of no practical importance. Urinary steroid excretion is still often measured and in this case an important point arises. Urinary excretion proceeds in slow pulses, probably reflecting reabsorption of biliary steroids from the gut and possibly renal handling of steroids. If the urine collections are made over reasonably long periods of time, 24 or 48 h, these pulses are evened out and the variability of urinary excretion approaches that of plasma concentration. But there is a great temptation to make do with shorter collection periods, like overnight urines. In this case the variability of urinary excretion obscures the significance of the measurement. It follows from the nature of steroid metabolism, and probably from creatinine metabolism also, that tricks such as using steroid-creatinine ratios are quite futile.

Homeostatic systems under feedback control exhibit small variations about a central mean, the so-called hunting phenomenon. The placenta is not subject to feedback control and does not exhibit a pulsatile release of its products. The variations in plasma concentration of its products are random and are probably connected with factors such as uterine blood flow which have nothing to do with biosynthesis or release. In general they are small, and hidden by the technical variation, although they may enhance or lessen the latter. Attempts to allow for likely physiological factors such as posture, activity or diet have not affected the variability of plasma oestriol concentration (Klopper et al. 1974).

Function

It is popularly assumed that naturally occurring substances exist for a purpose. In the case of trophoblast products this purpose is, in broad terms, adjustment of maternal physiology to yield the environment best suited to the survival of the fetoplacental unit. The specific roles proposed for the individual products will be listed in Chaps. 4–9 and can be divided into endocrine, metabolic and immunological functions.

Two general factors will be noted here: (1) the supposed functions of the trophoblast proteins are confined almost exclusively to the mother. The only exception known to us is the proposal (largely unproven) that placental hCG stimulates testosterone output by the fetal testis in mid trimester (Abramovich et al. 1974). It is very difficult to prove a case for fetal function with regard to the steroids, which are present in high concentration in the fetal circulation. Even in the mother many of the supposed functions of placental products are speculative rather than definitive, and it has even been suggested that the trophoblast products have no function whatsoever (Gordon and Chard 1979).

The latter is supported by some rare 'experiments of nature': the occasional pregnancy in which a specific product is almost totally deficient. Examples include placental sulphatase deficiency (leading to very low levels of oestriol), and deficiencies of hPL (Gaede et al. 1978) and SP1 (Grudzinskas et al. 1979). Pregnancies associated with these defects are usually entirely normal in every other respect, and it is difficult in the light of this evidence to suggest that these products serve any very essential biological role.

It is pertinent here to enquire how valid Diczfalusy's concept of a 'fetoplacental unit' really is. Certainly the fetus and its placenta is not an integrated unit with signals passing back and forth between the two, in the same sense as, say, the pituitary and the ovaries of the mother are a unit. They are a unit in the sense that much of the placental function is to provide the fetus with a controlled environment. The original description of the fetoplacental unit was in terms of oestrogen biosynthesis (Diczfalusy and Mancuso 1969). Later it was extended to cover many of the steroids shuttling back and forth between fetus and placenta. Steroids are synthesized by an array of enzymes, each responsible for a particular substituent on the molecule. Some enzymes, e.g. that which adds a hydroxyl group at C16 of the steroid nucleus, are present only in the fetal adrenal or liver. Other enzymes, e.g. the system which aromatises ring A of the nucleus, are present only in the placenta. Oestriol, which has both a C16 hydroxyl and an aromatised ring A, is therefore a true fetoplacental product. Whether its function lies with the fetus or the mother, or both, is not clear from the evidence currently available.

Control mechanisms

It has proved extremely difficult to demonstrate any mechanism which controls the production of any of the specific placental products. Where such a mechanism has been suggested (as for example the control of hPL release by maternal carbohydrates and lipids) the evidence is often disputed and subject to alternative explanations (Pavlou et al. 1973). We have proposed a hypothesis (Gordon and Chard 1979) which is susceptible to experimental study and not at variance with any of the accepted facts about placental synthesis. This hypothesis suggests that the potential for placental synthesis is a direct function of the total mass of the trophoblast, that the rate of release (and secondarily, of synthesis) is a function of the concentration of the substance in the maternal blood in the intervillous space, and that this, in turn depends on the rate of blood flow in the intervillous space (Fig. 2.2).

For proteins, synthesized in the trophoblast, this is an attractive hypothesis. When, however, the steroids are considered, new elements enter into the argument. At most the total mass of the trophoblast can exert only a remote secondary influence on steroidogenic steps in the fetus. Also the burden of steroids entering the maternal circulation carries a fraction of steroids which are simply being transmitted from fetal to maternal circulation, and are not at all subject to the processes which govern synthesis within the trophoblast. Finally substrate supply, from either mother or fetus, has a direct immediate effect on placental synthesis of some steroids, but no discernible effect on protein synthesis. Thus, injecting dehydroepiandrosterone sulphate into the maternal circulation can, in half an hour, quadruple the concentration of oestradiol in her veins; presumably as a result of increased placental utilisa-

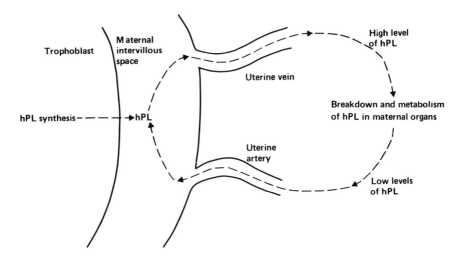

Fig. 2.2. Diagram to show how uteroplacental blood-flow may control the rate of synthesis by the trophoblast.

tion of this substrate. No amount of amino acids injected into the mother will make any significant difference to plasma hPL concentration.

Even in the case of the placental proteins this is not the easiest of concepts, and can perhaps be clarified by reference to a specific situation. Suppose that an equilibrium is set up with a constant amount of placental tissue, a constant rate of blood flow, and, therefore, a fixed concentration of a given placental protein in the blood. Now suppose that the blood flow is doubled. Almost immediately the concentration of the placental protein will halve because the same amount of product is now entering what is effectively twice the volume of blood. According to the hypothesis, the rate of release of the product will now increase until the concentration returns to its original level. At some time the rate of synthesis will also increase to meet the demand, and a new equilibrium will be established. The situation is analogous to that of dialysis of salts across a semi-permeable membrane; in a closed system solute will flow until the concentrations on the two sides of the membrane are equal; if the solvent on one side of the membrane is replaced solute will again flow until equilibrium is re-established.

Measurement

Measurement of the various products of the fetoplacental unit involves a very wide range of assay technologies. It is not the aim of this book to describe details of laboratory methodology, but some criteria are pertinent to the choice of a test for clinical use.

The most important point can be summarised in a few words: the better the test methodology, the better will be the clinical use of the test. This may seem obvious, even trite, but it is not often appreciated that this fact may be the sole feature determining the choice of one test over another. In most diagnostic biochemistry a substance is measured because it gives unique information about a patient. For example, corticotrophin (ACTH) is measured in many forms of endocrine pathology, despite the fact that the estimation is often imprecise, time consuming and expensive. But there is no alternative; no other measurement (e.g. of cortisol) will give exactly the same information. By contrast, estimation of many of the trophoblast products will give identical clinical results. Under these circumstances the choice can be determined by the relative merits of the different test methodologies. If compound x yields the same clinical results as compound y, and x is easier to measure, then measuring x is the better test.

There are a number of criteria by which any method for measuring a placental product may be judged (or any other biochemical parameter for that matter).

Sensitivity. This refers to the least amount of material which can be measured by the test. Generally sensitivity is an important criterion only in early pregnancy, when the concentration of placental products in blood or urine is low. In practice this applies above all to studies on abortion or the diagnosis of pregnancy. A common deception about sensitivity is often practised on the unwary: to give the absolute amount of material above zero which the test can detect. The clinician in a real-life situation is concerned only, having taken as much blood or urine from the patient as he reasonably can, with what is the smallest amount of product in that fluid that he can measure. The practical description of sensitivity is the least amount of material which can be discriminated from zero, in say, 10 ml of blood. A useful corollary is to determine by what stage of pregnancy such amounts are generally present.

Precision. How nearly will repeated estimations of the same sample give the same answer? The simplest technique is to measure a number of aliquots from the same sample. The precision is then represented by the standard deviation about the mean value. If the standard deviation is expressed as a percentage of the mean (coefficient of variation) it is independent of the absolute values and can be used to compare the precision of measurement of one product with that of another. When replicates are measured in a single batch they vary less than when measured in separate tests of the same sample. A reasonable intra-assay precision for most RIA procedures is 8%–10%. The equivalent figure for inter-assay measurements is 10%–12%.

Specificity. This refers to the capacity of a test to measure only the material it purports to measure and not to be influenced, positively or negatively, by any other. Many chemical tests have non-specific measuring end points and depend for their specificity on the purity of the final product presented to the measuring mechanism. The pendulum has swung far in the opposite direction with many immunoassay procedures. Antibodies, and to a lesser extent receptor or carrier proteins, will recognise with exquisite discrimination only the particular antigen for which they are programmed. As a rule it is sufficient proof of specificity to establish that the binding protein will not recognise a variety of related antigens.

Accuracy. This refers to how near to a known amount a test value is. This is simply determined by the percentage recovery of a known amount of material added to the fluid in which the measurements are usually made. Often it is difficult to get such fluids free of the endogenous product and accuracy has to be determined by first measuring the endogenous content of the fluid and then adding a known amount of material to it. In the case of placental products, male or non-pregnant female fluids which contain at most a trace of the material being measured, are adequate.

Convenience. This is a criterion composed of several elements. Firstly speed; generally clinicians want the result of a placental function test the same day. A test which takes a week to do is of no use to them. Secondly expense, which is compounded of the cost of materials and instruments and the number of tests. Thirdly skill; many assays which have nothing to recommend them but simplicity have enjoyed a great vogue.

Progress in diagnostic medicine is almost invariably by advances in laboratory technology rather than advances in fundamental clinical science. Most of the popular routine tests were introduced because the method became available and not necessarily because of some preconceived idea that the test would be valuable. This is well illustrated by the placental function tests. The concept of clinical measurement of chemical products of the fetus probably occurred to numerous people in the late 19th or early 20th century. However, it was the introduction of appropriate technology for steroid measurement in urine in the 1940s which led to the introduction of clinical tests in the 1950s. At that time alternatives to urinary steroids were conceptually obvious but technologically impossible; only the introduction of RIAs in the late 1960s and the 1970s was able to broaden the range of possibilities.

Trophoblast products in relation to obstetric pathology

With the exception of congenital abnormalities and simple mechanical problems, the fetus does not die of primary fetal 'disease'. The fetus dies, or is seriously damaged, because it is denied the materials on which it is totally dependent, and this deprivation arises in the placenta. All other defects, whether in the mother or the child, are secondary to placental pathology and it is therefore unfortunate that the placenta itself is so rarely the subject of routine pathological study. When pathologists do comment upon placentas it is often to observe on phenomena known to occur very commonly in perfectly normal pregnancies (e.g. the presence of infarcts and calcification). Little advantage has been taken of the excellent background information on this subject. We shall be obliged from time to time to use the term 'placental insufficiency' while recognising that this designation may be scientifically unsatisfactory. It is taken to include all those factors which may lead to a reduction in placental transfer of nutrients and waste products between mother and fetus and thus cause some of the fetal complications shown in Table 1.1. The term is very convenient in the context of placental function tests because it rather accurately describes the conditions under which these may give abnormal results.

It is worthwhile to consider briefly how the known forms of placental pathology might affect the output of trophoblast products. Various structures may be involved (Fig. 2.3) and will be discussed in turn.

The fetal capillaries

The synthetic functions of the trophoblast do not appear to depend on the integrity of the fetal circulation. Death of the fetus in the absence of placental pathology (e.g. congenital abnormalities, cord accidents) does not immediately affect the output of most trophoblast-specific products. It will, however, affect the synthesis of those products (e.g. oestriol) which depend upon fetal precursors.

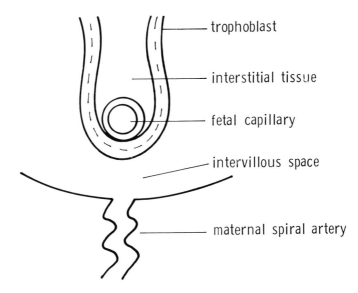

Fig. 2.3. The structures which may be affected by fetoplacental pathology and thus affect placental production.

The interstitial tissue of the chorionic villus

Oedema of the villous interstitial tissue is associated with fetal hydrops. This may lead to impairment of fetomaternal exchange and thus to a reduction in placental synthesis of materials which depend on fetal precursors. On its own, however, it would not cause a decrease in specific placental products.

The trophoblast basement membrane

Thickening of the basement membrane is associated with a number of pregnancy disorders, including pre-eclampsia, hypertension, diabetes mellitus and rhesus incompatibility (Fox 1978). The biochemical effects of this would be similar to those of other lesions on the fetal side of the trophoblast.

The trophoblast

Almost by definition, damage to the trophoblast will lead to a reduction in its synthetic function. Degeneration of the trophoblast (clumping of nuclei, fibrinoid deposition and thickening of the basement membrane) is associated with pre-eclampsia and hypertension. The reverse of this process is seen in the hypertrophy associated with rhesus iso-immunisation and maternal diabetes mellitus and appears to be specific to these conditions; the excessive mass of the trophoblast is reflected by elevated levels of specific placental products.

The intervillous space

Obstruction of the intervillous space invariably leads to death of the adjacent trophoblast and cessation of synthetic and transfer functions. Fibrin deposition in this site is a feature common to most forms of placental pathology, and varies from a thin layer on certain areas of the trophoblast (a normal finding in the term placenta) (Fox 1978) to the complete obliteration of the intervillous space which accompanies placental infarction. As with thrombus formation in other areas, the basic cause may be an alteration in the blood, change in blood flow (stasis), or damage to adjacent tissues. Any or all of these might be operative in complications of late pregnancy.

The maternal blood vessels

Changes in the maternal decidual arterioles may be the primary lesion leading to placental damage associated with diseases of pregnancy such as pre-eclampsia (Robertson et al. 1975). Minor degrees of obstruction at this site will lead to an overall reduction in uteroplacental bloodflow, with consequent decrease in both synthesis and transfer at the trophoblast. Major or total obstruction will lead to thrombus formation in the intervillous space and destruction of the trophoblast; assuming a localised lesion the fetal circulation may survive for a time but will serve no functional role.

References

Abramovich DR, Baker TG, Neal P (1974) Effect of human chorionic gonadotrophin on testosterone secretion by the foetal human testis in organ culture. J Endocrinol 60: 179
Burgos MH, Rodriguez EM (1966) Specialised zones in the trophoblast of the human term placenta. Am J Obstet Gynecol 96: 342
Diczfalusy E (1962) Endocrinology of the fetus. Acta Obstet Gynecol Scand 41 [Suppl 1]: 45
Diczfalusy E, Mancuso S (1969) Oestrogen metabolism in pregnancy. In Klopper A, Diczfalusy E (eds) Foetus and placenta. Blackwells, Oxford, pp 191-148
Fox H (1978) Pathology of the placenta, Saunders, London
Gaede P, Trolle D, Pedersen H (1978) Extremely low placental lactogen hormone values in an otherwise uneventful pregnancy. Acta Obstet Gynecol, Scand 57: 203
Gau G, Chard T (1976) Localisation of protein hormones of the placenta by immunoperoxidase techniques. Br J Obstet Gynaecol 83: 876
Gordon YB, Chard T (1979) The specific proteins of the human placenta: Some new hypotheses. In Klopper A, Chard T (eds) Placental proteins. Springer, Berlin, Heidelberg, New York, pp 1–21
Grudzinskas JG, Gordon YB, Humphreys JD, Brudenell M, Chard T (1979) Circulating levels of pregnancy specific β_1-glycoprotein in pregnancies complicated by diabetes mellitus. Br J Obstet Gynaecol. 86: 978

References

Klopper A (1972) Estriol in amniotic fluid. Am J Obstet Gynecol. 112: 459
Klopper A, Wilson G, Masson G (1974) The variability of plasma hormone levels in late pregnancy. In Scholler R (ed) Hormonal investigations in human pregnancy. Sepe, Paris, pp 77-76
Klopper A, Smith R, Davidson I (1979) The measurement of trophoblast proteins as a test of placental function. In: Klopper A, Chard T (eds) Placental proteins. Springer, Berlin, Heidelberg, New York, pp 23–42
Ludwig H (1974) Surface structure of the human placenta. In: Moghissi KS, Hafez ESE (eds) The placenta: Biological and clinical aspects. Thomas, Springfield, pp 40–64
Panigel M (1974) Relation of the ultrastructure of the placenta to its function. In: Moghissi KS, Hafez ESE (eds) The placenta: Biological and clinical aspects. Thomas, Springfield, pp 5–39
Pavlou C, Chard T, Landon J, Letchworth AT (1973) Circulating levels of human placental lactogen in late pregnancy: The effect of glucose loading, smoking, and exercise. Eur J Obstet. Gynaecol. Reprod Biol 34: 45
Robertson WB, Brosens I, Dixon G (1975) Uteroplacental vascular pathology. Eur J Obstet. Gynaecol. Reprod. Biol 5: 47

Chapter 3
Analysis of the Clinical Results of Placental Function Tests

It is now apparent from basic principles (Chap. 2) that measurement of fetoplacental products in the mother might be a useful parameter of the overall function of fetus or placenta. The question that this chapter will address is 'how useful?'. Though superficially simple, this question has given rise to more arguments and doubts than any other aspect of the subject. The doubts have arisen from the failure to appreciate that few tests in diagnostic medicine give absolute results: instead, there is almost always an overlap between normal and abnormal, and the information given is in terms of relative risk rather than certainty. For example, a normal result of a biochemical test cannot guarantee that the outcome of a pregnancy will be normal: there is no way in which it would be expected to predict mechanical problems during labour. Similarly, it is self-evident that the description of a 'normal range' (see below) must be based on statistical limits which will exclude some subjects at the extremes of the range. 'Abnormal' results must, therefore, include some normal subjects and, again, cannot guarantee an abnormal outcome.

In this chapter we will discuss the definitions of normality and abnormality in obstetric care, and the means by which it is possible to judge the clinical efficiency of *any* parameter, with special reference to the biochemical tests.

Definition of normality

The establishment of a normal range is widely agreed to be the basic requirement for the evaluation and application of a test of fetal wellbeing. Superficially the definition of a normal pregnancy should be relatively simple, and it is usually achieved by specifying a series of exclusions, for example, "the criteria for a normal pregnancy were delivery of a single infant in good condition between 38–42 weeks by dates, with fetal weight of 2.5 kg or greater and with no maternal complications, e.g. pre-eclampsia, antepartum haemorrhage, rhesus incompatibility, essential hypertension, or diabetes mellitus". On closer inspection, however, this apparently simple definition can be faulted on a number of counts.

The first and most obvious concerns details of the criteria used. For instance, should an arbitrary lower limit be given for normal fetal weight (2.5 kg) or should a more specific figure be used, based on the limits from another and larger study such as that of the British Perinatal Mortality Survey (Butler and Bonham 1963)? Should more details be given of the complications, and of fetal condition at delivery? Should it be specified that the group included only those patients who were certain of their dates? Should account have been taken of whether the labour was spontaneous or induced? Should parity be considered?

The second problem concerns the clinical usefulness of a normal range based on the above criteria, all of which are retrospective, i.e. they depend on a knowledge of the outcome of the pregnancy which is available to the scientific investigator but is not available to the clinician at the time that he sees the patient. The clinician is faced with an individual patient who is still pregnant, not a population all of whom have delivered. He will not be able to classify the patient on any of the criteria set out, with the possible exception of single or multiple pregnancy. He does not know that the child will be delivered alive, when it will be delivered, how much it will weigh once delivered, or if a complication is not already present, whether it may not occur at a later stage. There can be no logical reason for excluding from a normal range any of those factors of which the clinican might be unaware at the time that the sample is taken. We would argue that the obstetrician would be better served by a range which embraces the whole of the population which he serves (Fig. 3.1); that this range be divided into levels specifying different degrees of fetal risk (Fig 3.2); and that alternative ranges should only be used when a clinical parameter such as diabetes provides a definitive and prospective indication of the selection of a subpopulation.

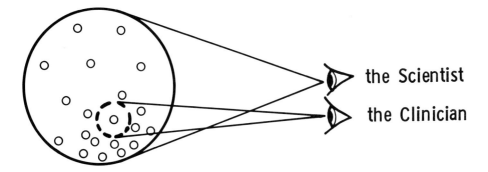

Fig. 3.1. The problems of research on biochemical tests of fetal wellbeing. Both scientist, and clinician are looking at a universe of individuals. The scientist, working retrospectively, can see the whole universe and notes that there is a cluster of individuals in one part of the universe. The clinician can only see a single individual and will not realise that this individual is part of the cluster unless he has good communication with the scientist.

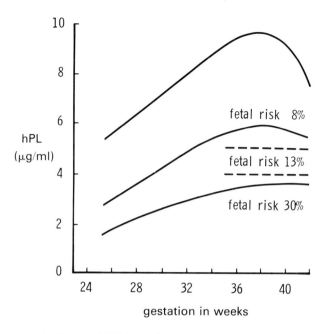

Fig. 3.2. Maternal hPL levels in an unselected obstetric population. The mean ± two standard deviations (after log transform) are shown, together with the fetal risk associated with different ranges.

Definition of abnormality

As with normality, the definition of abnormality appears simple, but problems can arise at two levels: first in specifying the nature and degree of the abnormality; second, in specifying the manner in which a biochemical parameter might assist in the clinical management of the abnormality.

Failure to provide an adequate definition of abnormality is very common in the literature on tests of fetal wellbeing. For example, a group of diabetics may be presented without reference to the severity of the condition, or whether the condition is established or gestational. A similar situation exists with pre-eclampsia (a condition which has almost as many definitions as there are workers in the field). The 'mild' variety (patients with a maximum diastolic blood pressure between 90 and 99 mmHg) can present particular difficulty, because of the frequency with which readings in this range are found during labour in patients who have no other perinatal complications. Probably the major problem arises with the definition of 'intrauterine growth retardation' (synonyms 'small-for-dates', 'light-for-dates', 'dysmaturity'). Although this condition is occasionally identified on the basis of detailed paediatric study of the neonate, most commonly the diagnosis is based on the

Definition of abnormality

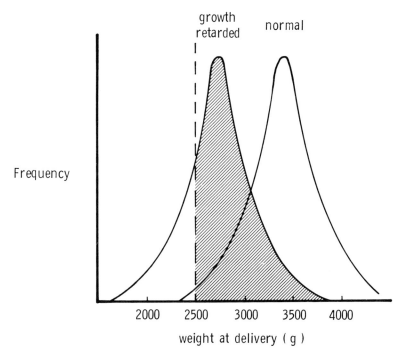

Fig. 3.3. The 'submerged two-thirds' of intrauterine growth retardation. On the right, the frequency distribution of delivered weight for normal pregnancy. On the left, the frequency distribution of delivered weight for growth-retarded fetuses, assuming a mean reduction of 650 g from their potential 'normal' weight. On this assumption, the shaded area shows those cases of growth retardation (about two-thirds of the total) which will fail to be diagnosed on the basis of an arbitrary cut-off point at 2500 g.

delivered weight of the child, and the relation of this to the normal range for the stage of gestation. Useful though this may be as a practical definition, it has the disadvantage that it must exclude a substantial proportion of growth-retarded neonates. Thus, delivered weight must reflect the genetic growth potential of the fetus, and variation in this leads to the observed distribution of birth weight in normal pregnancies. Growth retardation implies the operation of some factor which inhibits achievement of this potential, and it must be assumed that this factor may apply to any fetus of any growth potential. The reduction in potential weight which can be described as pathological has been estimated at 653 g (Ounsted and Ounsted 1973). Using this figure a range can be constructed for the delivered weights of growth-retarded infants (Fig. 3.3). The overlap between this range and the normal range leads to the conclusion that only some 30% of growth-retarded babies will be identified as such on the basis of weight at birth. This conclusion is well supported by available evidence on mortality rates for children whose birth weight is in the range of normal (Fig. 3.4).

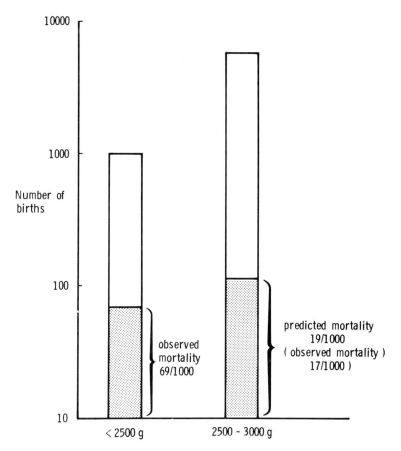

Fig. 3.4. The possible importance of the 'submerged two-thirds' of intrauterine growth retardation, assuming that this is a major factor in perinatal mortality. The observed mortality rate for neonates weighing less than 2500 g is about 69 per 1000 (*left hand column*); this group represents some 2.5% of the population. The group 2500 – 3000 g includes some 15% of the population, and is shown in proportion (*right hand column*). This group will include 50% of the growth-retarded fetuses; for the number of births shown this would lead to a total of 115 deaths, or a mortality rate of 19 per 1000. The observed mortality rate is 17 per 1000, which is remarkably close to the figure predicted by this model.

A further problem is to specify the manner in which a biochemical parameter can be of clinical value. To state that the levels of a given hormone are reduced in, for example, pre-eclampsia, may be of considerable academic interest. In itself, however, this does not help the clinician since the diagnosis of pre-eclampsia will in no sense depend on biochemical findings. It could well be that the overall levels are low, but provide no distinction between cases in which the fetus is at particular risk and those in which it is not. Unless the test can give such information to the clinician, it is of little or no value. A further point arising from this concerns the use of a range for the condition as the clinical yardstick, rather than a normal range. This is particularly well illustrated by hPL measurements in diabetic pregnancies (Chap. 6). The overall levels of hPL are increased in this condition; with a specific element of fetal risk they are reduced, but only relative to the range of diabetics. If compared with the normal range the 'risk' levels are not apparently of any prognostic significance. On occasion, however, as will be seen that PAPP-A and PP5, placental function tests can give prognostic information about specific complications.

Following the arguments presented above, it is obvious that claims for the value of any test in the diagnosis of intrauterine growth retardation should be examined with care. A parameter which is related to delivered weight clearly has intrinsic merit, since this is information which cannot necessarily be obtained by other means. However, low birth weight does not inevitably indicate growth retardation, while a 'normal' weight might be compatible with this diagnosis. For this reason an important criterion, rarely, if ever, applied in practice, is whether the test can distinguish the small baby which is growth retarded and carries a high risk, from the small baby which is otherwise normal and carries low risk. At the present time there is no strong evidence that the placental function tests provide information which goes beyond the simple relation to mass.

Numerical definition of the normal range

Regardless of how a normal range is defined (whether as a total population, or on more restricted criteria of normality) it still has to be described by a set of numbers. Several methods of description have been used; these include the use of simple absolute limits; the use of the Gaussian (normal) distribution, with or without transformation; and the non-parametric approach (median and centiles and multiples of the median). Overall, the latter is probably the most satisfactory at the present time because none of the biochemical parameters of placental function have a Gaussian distribution of normal values, however normality is defined.

Absolute limits

This is the simplest approach, and merely sets the limits as the highest and lowest numbers observed experimentally. The great disadvantage is that sooner or later values will be obtained in apparently normal pregnancies which lie at the extremes of the statistical distribution. Limits set by such values will include virtually the whole obstetric population, normal or pathological, thereby rendering the range useless for clinical purposes.

Gaussian (normal) distribution

In the past, this has been much the commonest way of describing the normal range. It assumes that the values follow the classic bell-shaped Gaussian (or normal) frequency distribution, and can therefore be described by the mean plus or minus standard deviations; two standard deviations above the mean to two standard deviations below the mean embraces 95% of all normal values. This approach has the great advantage that meaningful limits can be established on the basis of a relatively small set of numbers (20 or more observations are usually adequate). The disadvantage, which is quite over-riding and negates much of the value of the earlier literature on this subject, is that all placental function tests (and for that matter, most of the other numerical parameters measured in biomedicine) do not follow a straightforward Gaussian distribution, and limits generated by this analysis give a false picture of the 'real' distribution (Fig. 3.5).

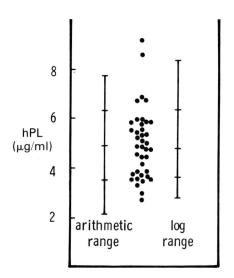

Fig. 3.5. Skewed distribution of placental lactogen (hPL) values from a normal range for the 34th week of pregnancy. When means and standard deviations are calculated in arithmetic from the resulting statistical range is a poor fit to the observed spread of results. When the same calculation is made after logarithmic transformation, the resulting range is a much closer fit. It is likely that skewed distributions of this type will apply to the majority of biological parameters, including all hormonal tests of fetal wellbeing.

Transformed Gaussian distribution

It is now widely accepted that any set of biological results which can be described on a numerical scale running from zero upwards will show a skewed distribution, because the results are weighted by the occurrence of a few relatively high values. This yields an artefactual increase in the arithmetic mean, with more observations below it than above it.

As a matter of empirical observation, sets of results of this type will approximate to a Gaussian distribution if they are analysed after logarithmic or square root transformation. In other words, each number is converted to its log or square root, means and standard deviations calculated, and the limits so derived converted back by taking antilogarithms or squares. This procedure is illustrated in Fig. 3.5, which also demonstrates that the results can be a much better 'fit' to the real data.

Non-parametric distribution (median and centiles)

This approach makes no assumption whatsoever about the distribution of values, and is equally descriptive of a classic Gaussian curve or a set of results which are distributed completely at random. Thus, the *median* is that value which divides a population into two equal halves, even though the lower half may range from 5 to 10 and the upper half from 10 to a million. A similar argument applies to centiles: for example, the 10th centile is that value below which 10% of the population lies. This type of analysis is particularly appropriate to studies where the normal range is based on a total population rather than on an arbitrary selection of 'normals'.

The absence of any assumptions is a major advantage of the non-parametric approach which in our opinion makes it the method of choice for the description of ranges of placental function tests. However, it has two disadvantages, neither of which is fundamental. The first is the fact that definition of the more extreme centiles (broadly speaking, less then the 10th or more than the 90th) becomes very inaccurate unless there is a fairly substantial data-base. Thus, for example, it would not be possible to give a meaningful estimate of the 99th centile if only 20 values were available, whereas it would be possible to estimate 3 or 4 standard deviations. But since the commonly used limits are the 10th or 5th centiles, this does not place exceptional demands for the generation of data. Second, tests of 'statistical significance' are more difficult to carry out on non-parametric data than on normally distributed data; 'difficult', in this context, means that they cannot readily be performed on a hand-held calculator. With the advent of inexpensive microcomputers this is no longer a problem.

Multiples of the median

This is a variation of the non-parametric approach which to some extent solves the problem of defining extremes given a small data-base. A reasonably accurate median can be obtained from small numbers, and a multiple of this (e.g. 0.5 × median; 2.5 × median) will be equally accurate. Providing a good estimate of the appropriate multiple is available (e.g. from the published data-base of a group which has examined very large numbers of samples) then a new group can establish stable limits on the basis of relatively small numbers of results. This method has been applied very successfully to the use of alphafetoprotein measurements in the diagnosis of neural tube defects of the fetus. It deserves more attention in the context of the placental function tests.

Routine use of normal ranges

Fortunately, the routine clinical use of placental function tests demands no basic understanding of the arguments set out above. All that is required by the clinician is a simple statement of what the limits are. However, he should be reassured that the limits he uses have been set by someone with a good understanding of the arguments, otherwise there will be endless confusion and disappointment. Furthermore, he should be prepared to supply the laboratory, if a new test is set up, with enough samples to ensure that useful limits can be established. In the next section we will propose a relatively straightforward exercise by which any group (i.e. clinician plus laboratory) can both establish its own limits and judge the clinical efficiency of a test in a local context.

How useful is a test? Analysis of clinical efficiency

Perhaps the main advance in placental function testing in the past 5 years has not been in the discovery of new substances or the discovery of new ways of measuring old substances, but in the exploitation of new methods of data analysis. It is now possible (and should soon become universal in the literature) to present studies in such a way that they can be directly compared with other similar studies, or studies on another test, or even studies on some totally different parameter. The key to understanding these lies in a familiarity with the sets of terms shown in Tables 3.1 and 3.2.

True and false positives and negatives

The definition of these terms is shown in Table 3.1. Though their derivation is fairly obvious, it may be helpful to consider a specific example.

A new placental function test is available. One hundred pregnant women are selected[1] and a blood sample is taken at 36 weeks' gestation. The test substance is measured and the weight of the child[2] at delivery is noted.

The values of the test results and delivered weights are ranked (i.e. arranged in ascending order of magnitude) and the median and 10th centiles[3]

---

[1] The nature of the selection process is not particularly important. For this study it may well include any mixture of normals and abnormals, though a random choice (e.g. 100 successive patients) would be preferable. One hundred subjects is probably the minimum necessary.

[2] Delivered weight is the most common clinical parameter examined in relation to placental function tests. Other parameters (e.g. fetal distress neonatal asphyxia) could equally well be added.

[3] The 10th centile has been chosen for this exercise, though any other centile could be examined if appropriate.

Table 3.1. The definition of true and false positives, and true and false negatives

True positive (TP): the level of the test substances is low[a] in the presence of the clinical abnormality[b].

True negative (TN): the level of the test substances is normal in the absence of the clinical abnormality.

False positive (FP): the level of the test substance is low in the absence of the clinical abnormality.

False negative (FN): the level of the test substances is normal in the presence of the clinical abnormality.

[a]'Low' means below some predetermined limit: in the case of the example shown in Table 3.2 this is the 10th centile for the whole range of substance X.

[b]In the example shown in Tables 3.2 and 3.3 the abnormality (growth retardation) is also defined by reference to a set of ranked numbers. The same procedure can be applied to a non-numerical 'yes-no' situation, e.g. the presence or absence of fetal distress.

Table 3.2. The definition of sensitivity, specificity and predictive value (TP, TN, etc. are defined in Table 3.1). The numbers given are from a hypothetical study involving the measurement of substance X in a population of 100 patients. Low levels of substance X (less than the 10th centile of the whole range) are examined for their relationship to intrauterine growth retardation (delivered weight less than the 10th centile of the population examined). These data are further analysed in Table 3.3. and commented upon in the text.

Sensitivity	$(\frac{TP}{TP + FN})$	$\frac{5}{5 + 5}$	= 50%
Specificity	$(\frac{TN}{FP + TN})$	$\frac{85}{5 + 85}$	= 94.4%
Predictive value	$(\frac{TP}{FP + TP})$	$\frac{5}{5 + 5}$	= 50%

are calculated for both sets of data (this procedure can easily be done manually but is greatly helped by access to even the smallest computer). The numbers of true and false positives, and true and false negatives, are then estimated according to the definitions of Table 3.1.

At this stage a preliminary inspection of the data may show if the test is of value. Thus, if the number of true positives were 1, it would be immediately apparent that this is the number expected if the test result is completely independent of fetal weight; if the number of true positives were 10 the test would be perfect and bias should be suspected. More commonly the number will lie between 1 and 10 and the statistical significance of the association can be assessed by the Chi-square test (Tables 3.2, 3.3).

The data generated on positive and negative results can be used to calculate sensitivity, specificity and predictive value.

Table 3.3. Assessing the statistical significance of a set of observations on a test carried out on 100 patients. The numbers are from the hypothetical study shown in Table 3.2. The reader is advised to consult a text book of statistics for more detailed information on the construction of these tables.

	Observed frequency (O)	Expected frequency (E)[a]	(O−E)[b]	(O−E)$^{2/E}$
True negatives	85	81	3.5	0.15
False negatives	5	9	−3.5	1.36
False positives	5	9	−3.5	1.36
True positives	5	1	3.5	12.5
	100	100	0	15.12 = Chi-square[c]

[a] I.e. the frequency expected if the two observations (substance X and fetal weight) were completely independent.
[b] This figure has had Yates correction applied.
[c] This value of Chi-square would be a highly significant association.

Sensitivity, specificity and predictive value

These terms are defined in Table 3.2, and the concepts of sensitivity and predictive value are shown diagramatically in Fig. 3.6.

Because the terms are not universally familiar it is worthwhile to expand on their exact clinical meaning 'Sensitivity' is an index of the proportion of all cases of the clinical abnormality which is associated with abnormal levels of the test substance. 'Specificity' is an index of the proportion of all patients with normal levels of the test substance who also have normal infants. 'Predictive value' is an index of the proportion of all patients with abnormal levels of the test substance who also have the clinical abnormality.

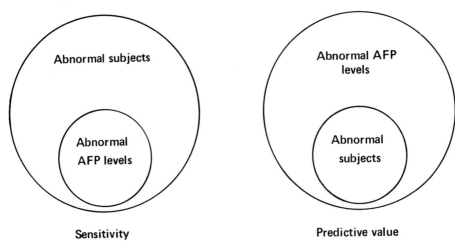

Fig. 3.6. A diagrammatic illustration of the concepts of 'sensitivity' and 'predictive value' of a clinical test. *AFP*, alphafetoprotein.

Predictive value is the key number for the clinician faced with an individual patient. In the hypothetical study described in Table 3.2, low levels of substance X would tell him that the patient had a 50% risk of intrauterine growth retardation. Sensitivity and specificity are not relevant to the individual patient, but can dictate the choice of test in the first instance. A sensitivity of 50% (Table 3.2), as against the random figure of 10% if the test were of no value at all, suggests that the test is highly efficient.

The relative risk ratio

Relative risk is defined as the ratio of the percentage of positives which are true positives to the percentage of negatives which are false negatives (TP/TP + FP:FN/FN + TN). Though not the easiest concept to grasp in words, it effectively produces a single figure by which the overall value of a test may be judged and compared with other parameters including non-biochemical tests. A relative risk ratio of 1 indicates that the observation does not distinguish a risk which is any different from that in the population as a whole; below 1 the observation indicates a reduced risk, above 1 an increased risk.

Other aspects of the analysis of placental function tests

Variation in the parameter measured

The importance of time-to-time variation in individual subjects, and of the variation due to the method of measurement, have already been discussed. Another very important variable is that between individuals—the fact that babies and their mothers vary in size. Variation of this type represents an irreducible minimum which cannot be influenced by the investigator, except perhaps by the judicious selection of groups. For the sort of test dealt with in this book it seems likely that the minimum possible variation will be equivalent to that of fetal or placental weight, i.e. around 15%.

Design of studies on tests of fetal wellbeing

Several important criticisms can be levelled at many of the studies purporting to show the value of one or the other biochemical test of fetal wellbeing. Prominent among these criticisms are that the study has been carried out on insufficient numbers of patients and samples, and that it is all too often based on a selected group of patients, the results from whom have been analysed in isolation from the population of which they were part. Some of the difficulties arising from the retrospective analysis of selected groups have already been discussed above. The purpose of this section is to consider the optimal design of such investigations.

There can be no question that the best possible design is a prospective survey on a complete population. A 'population' in this sense may be derived from a single antenatal clinic, or all the antenatal clinics of a given hospital, or even several hospitals within a district. The basic requirement is that it should embrace all patients, without any exclusions, in a group whose initial selection is essentially random. The plan of the experiment is simple: every patient has a blood sample collected at every antenatal visit. Exceptions can be made only for those subjects in whom venepuncture is extremely difficult, or who refuse the procedure.

The over-riding advantage of this design is that it permits analysis of results in the context in which they initially present to the clinician. In other words, it does not yield only isolated groups of normals and abnormals judged on retrospective criteria. From the point of view of the statistician, it presents a large volume of data, indeed, the most complete set of data which can be achieved within the practical limits of antenatal care. The data can be analysed either serially, or as single samples from a given week of gestation. Finally, and in contrast to most other plans of investigation, it permits retrospective analysis of levels before the onset of specific complications, an analysis which is not possible with the selective approach.

The disadvantages of a prospective survey are as follows: (1) a high degree of organisation and co-operation is necessary at the clinical level; (2) resistance might be encountered from patients; in practice, and provided the nature of the procedure is explained at the booking clinic, this is very unusual; (3) the method of measurement must be simple, reproducible and capable of a high throughput; there is no point in starting on a prospective survey with an assay which is not well established and continuously monitored with a quality control system; (4) a data retrieval system must be established, preferably one which permits easy transfer of information on to punched cards and magnetic tape; the decision of what information to record can be difficult—the commonest fault is too much rather than too little.

A fully prospective study of the type described above, while theoretically desirable, will invariably be time consuming and expensive. We now believe that excellent information can be obtained from the limited (but nevertheless well-designed) study proposed on p. 26, i.e. 100 randomly selected subjects at a fixed week of gestation, and comparison of test levels with clearly defined parameters of fetal outcome. This simple investigation does not permit an elaborate analysis of the place of the test in antenatal care. However, it does permit the generation of limits for clinical action, the comparison of similar tests, and a preliminary evaluation of whether a new[4] test is of clinical value in the context of its intended use.

---

[4]'New' may mean a completely new test substance, or a change in methodology for an existing substance, or the transfer of an existing test to a new environment.

Controlled studies on placental function tests

It is often, and correctly, insisted that a therapeutic or diagnostic measure should be subjected to controlled study before it is applied in routine clinical practice. For a test of fetal wellbeing it is relatively easy to show in retrospect that what was measured related to the outcome of the pregnancy. It is much more difficult to show how knowledge of the measurements would have affected the outcome of pregnancy. In the context of obstetrics, 'outcome' can be a rather diffuse term. Fetal distress and neonatal asphyxia are very much in the eye of the beholder; intrauterine growth retardation, even when identified, cannot be prevented. By contrast, fetal death is a quite unarguable entity, and may be prevented by early delivery. Thus, fetal mortality provides the simplest yardstick for the controlled study of a test: a population is divided randomly into two halves; in the one the results of the test are reported and acted upon; in the other the results are not reported. Does mortality differ between the two groups? At the present time there is only one such study, carried out on a prospective basis, in the entire literature of this subject (Spellacy et al. 1975) and it gives a clear-cut value to the determination of hPL levels. Other studies of this type would be of great interest. Inevitably, the number of patients will have to be large. For a population with a perinatal mortality of 25 per 1000, only 10 of these deaths will be attributable to factors which can be identified by biochemical measurements. Under these circumstances, a total of 1500 subjects would have to be studied to establish a difference between the groups significant at the 5% level, and 2700 subjects for significance at the 1% level.

Importance of serial determinations

One of the basic tenets of the literature on placental function tests is that serial observations are of more value than single observations. Traditionally, this is founded on the concept that falling values indicate a high degree of fetal risk. Less well recognised, though perhaps more important, is the fact that, regardless of the trend, a number of values give a better estimate than a single value of where an individual lies in relation to the population as a whole.

It is worthwhile to examine both these concepts in relation to the observations already made on assay variability, and also to time-to-time biological variation in an individual subject. The true extent of the changes which may occur, for solely non-pathological reasons, is often masked by the apparently favourable figures given for the inherent variation in a measured parameter. For example, implicit in a quoted day-to-day variation of 15% (a common estimate for some oestrogen determinations) is that a fall in serial levels of 30% could be quite compatible with a random change of no pathological significance. Furthermore, the figure of 15% is a mean and implies that even higher figures occur, with still greater random fluctuation. For materials showing high day-to-day variation, the reductio ad absurdum is that there is

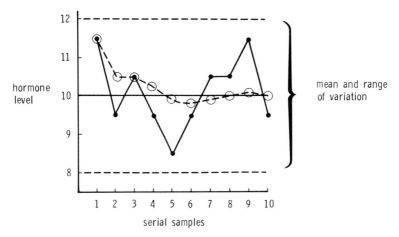

Fig. 3.7. The value of serial samples. The hormone measured has an overall variation of ± 20% and serial samples (●——●) show fluctuations within these limits. However, if the cumulative mean is calculated (○——○) the observed pattern stabilises when five or more serial results are available, thus providing a much better estimate of the real situation in an individual subject. It should be noted that this analysis would not apply if the hormone levels were showing a progressive rise or fall over the period studied; for example, serial levels of plasma oestriol at weekly intervals in late pregnancy.

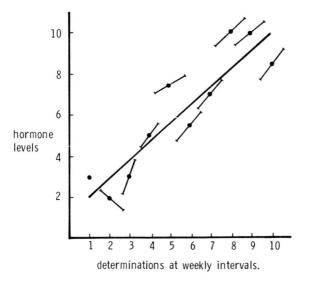

Fig. 3.8. The problem of drawing a regression line on serial and increasing hormone values from an individual subject. The continuous line shows the real trend of values. The points (●) show serial weekly determinations, assuming a coefficient of variation of about 20%, which includes assay error and day-to-day variation. The line through each point shows the slope of a 'least squares regression' based on that and the previous values. The calculated regression is at no point completely parallel to the 'real' trend; even after 10 weeks there is still a discrepancy which could be clinically misleading.

almost no change, however apparently large, that can be defined as abnormal.

The effect of cumulated values on the confidence estimates to the trend in an individual is illustrated in Fig. 3.7, and provides more than sufficient argument for the superiority of serial determinations. For measurement of blood samples, this does not necessarily indicate that the clinician should wait several days for the picture to be clarified: multiple determinations on the same samples, or serial samples collected over a period of hours, would have much the same effect, a concept of some importance which has been little used in clinical practice.

One group has studied the variation in oestriol levels at 5-min intervals, and concluded that serial samples collected in this manner yield a much more stable value for the individual than does the result of a single sample (Buster 1981). The practical problems of this approach can perhaps be overcome by the use of an indwelling needle for the multiple sampling, together with a single analysis of the pooled samples.

A further problem in the analysis of sequential biochemical determinations in pregnancy arises from the fact that levels may change continuously with respect to time. Under these circumstances, the logical procedure would be to fit a line to the serial points, and then to use this line to assess the relationship of the individual to the population. The difficulty with this approach is that a rather large number of points is needed before this line can be established with confidence (Fig. 3.8).

References

Buster JF (1981) Clinical applications of steroid assay tests of feto-placental function. In: Abraham GE (ed) Radioassay systems in clinical endocrinology. Marcel Dekker, New York, pp 349–371
Butler NR, Bonham DG (1963) Perinatal mortality. Livingstone, Edinburgh
Spellacy WN, Buhi WC, Birk SA (1975) The effectiveness of human placental lactogen measurements as an adjunct in decreasing perinatal deaths. J Obstet Gynecol. 121: 835

Chapter 4
Placental Enzymes

The human placenta contains a wide variety of enzymes, most of which represent the range of structural and metabolic enzymes found in all mammalian cells. Included among these are the enzymes responsible for placental synthesis of proteins and steroids, e.g. 3β-hydroxysteroid dehydrogenase. However, none of these distinguish the placenta from other endocrine tissues and as they are not 'exported' from the trophoblast there is no obvious change in their circulating levels.

By contrast, the serum levels of a number of hydrolytic enzymes increase substantially during pregnancy. From the very extensive literature on this subject (Hagerman 1969) it is not always clear whether such increases are the direct result of placental synthesis or whether the increases arise from other tissues. Futhermore, it is often uncertain whether a given enzyme activity defined in the placenta is specific to this organ (i.e. shows very striking qualitative or quantitative differences from tissues in the non-pregnant adult). However, there are some enzymes synthesised and secreted by the placenta which are, to all intents and purposes, specific. The most notable of these are heat-stable alkaline phosphatase (HSAP) and cystine aminopeptidase (CAP—also referred to as oxytocinase).

As specific products of the placental trophoblast, both HSAP and CAP are candidates for placental function tests. In the late 1960s and early 1970s there was a spate of reports to this effect but it is fair to state that such studies were limited in scope, frequently yielded unsatisfactory results, and that today estimation of enzymes is not widely used as a placental function test.

Chemistry, synthesis and metabolism

Alkaline phosphatase activity in serum appears as a number of so-called isoenzymes, differentiated by different rates of migration on electrophoresis. Some of these are unique to the placenta, which contains several genetically determined variants; these have the notable characteristic that their activity is resistant to heating at 50°–70°C. The molecular weight is approximately 116,000 daltons (Gottlieb and Sussman 1968). A similar but not quite identical isoenzyme is found in the blood and tissues of some cases of carcinoma, and is known as the 'Regan isoenzyme' after the patient in whom it was first discovered. Cystine aminopeptidase is a single molecular species with a molecular weight of 290,000, and an isoelectric point of 3.7.

Functions

The general functions of the alkaline phosphatases are concerned with active transport at the cell membrane level in a variety of tissues. In the circulation (pregnant or non-pregnant) no function has been proposed. CAP is a non-specific N-terminal endopeptidase, originally discovered by its destructive effect on oxytocin in vitro (and hence the name oxytocinase). However, the hypothesis that CAP protects the pregnant uterus against the activity of endogenous oxytocin, and that it might play an important part in the onset of labour, has never been proven; indeed, there is no evidence that the half-life of oxytocin differs between the pregnant and non-pregnant states.

Measurement

The placental enzymes are measured in serum by classic substrate conversion techniques with a spectrophotometric end point (Table 4.1). In the case of HSAP, serum is pre-treated by heating at 50°–70°C to inactivate the heat-labile form which is not specific to pregnancy.

Clinical enzyme measurement is fraught with problems (e.g. the requirement for exact conditions of ionic strength, pH, and temperature; the presence of non-specific inhibitory substances in serum samples). Unless the greatest care is taken these can lead to error, and we have already emphasised (Chap. 2) that a poor system of measurement may effectively wipe out the value of a test. This, rather than any inherent biological factor, is probably the reason why clinical experience with placental enzymes has been generally unfavourable. Furthermore, virtually every author on clinical application has used a slightly different method, making comparison difficult (Tables 4.2, 4.3).

Maternal levels in normal pregnancy

HSAP and CAP in maternal blood show a progressive increase during pregnancy (see references to Tables 4.2 and 4.3). Insofar as can be inter-

Table 4.1. Measurement of HSAP and CAP in pregnancy serum

Enzyme	Substrate
CAP	L-cystine bis-p-nitroanilide dihydrobromide[a]
HSAP	Disodium phenyl phosphate[b]

[a]Other substances have been used, some of which were rejected on the grounds of carcinogenicity.
[b]Numerous variations have been described, chiefly in the time and temperature for pre-incubation of the sample.

preted from the rather confusing evidence, the pattern of increase would seem to be the sigmoid curve characteristic of most trophoblastic products.

Clinical application of HSAP and CAP measurement in maternal serum

The literature on the clinical application of HSAP and CAP measurements is very limited and most was written at a time when rigorous criteria for the clinical efficiency of a placental function test were not available. For example, some workers presented individual cases in the absence of a normal range, and clear definition of the clinical abnormality (such as the delivered weight of the child) was often lacking. We have, therefore, chosen to present the data in the very non-specific and discursive form of Tables 4.2 and 4.3. The only unusual aspect of these data is the claim, as yet unconfirmed, that *elevated* HSAP levels are of diagnostic value (Merrett and Hunter 1973). The principle would be similar to that in which other damaged tissues (e.g. heart muscle) release intracellular enzymes, measurement of which can be of great diagnostic value.

Table 4.2. Clinical studies on the use of maternal HSAP determinations

Authors	Conclusion
Elder 1971	'Serum HSAP levels are probably of no value in the prediction of a small for dates baby.'
Curzen and Southcombe 1970	'Significant... correlation... between... serum HSAP level and crude placental weight.'
Merrett and Hunter 1973	'... a raised HSAP level can often be indicative of some present, past, or future abnormality in the patient.'
Curzen and Varma 1971	'Serum HSAP determinations were found to be of no use in predicting fetal distress, the Apgar score at birth, or fetal dysmaturity.'
Shane and Suzuki 1974[a]	'... no reliable range in placental alkaline phosphatase values in normal pregnancy... no usable trend of values... no correlation... with birthweight.'

[a]This reference includes an excellent review of the subject.

Table 4.3. Clinical studies on the use of maternal serum CAP estimation

Authors	Conclusion
Tovey 1969	'Serum oxytocinase estimations have been found to be of considerable help in complicated pregnancies.'
Watson et al. 1973	'Five foeto-placental function tests were studied... plasma cystine aminopeptidase was the least sensitive indicator of foetoplacental dysfunction.'
Hensleigh and Krantz 1970	'... good correlation between sequential maternal serum CAP activity and the clinical and pathologic findings of placental insufficiency.'

Very broadly, the following conclusions may be reached: measurement of HSAP has been almost universally rejected as a placental function test (Table 4.2); measurement of CAP has had its proponents but the published evidence for its value is very limited in scope (Table 4.3).

Other placental enzymes of potential clinical interest

Three placental enzymes, although not measurable in peripheral maternal blood, are nevertheless of some clinical interest. The first of these is arylsulphatase. The oestrogens in the fetal circulation, particularly oestriol, are mainly present as sulphates. Such sulphates are not lipid soluble and traverse the placental barrier very slowly. The transfer of oestriol from fetus to mother is greatly facilitated by placental arylsulphatase, which hydrolyses the oestrogen sulphates presenting from the fetal circulation and thus permits secretion of the free steroid into the maternal circulation. The clinical interest in this enzyme springs from the fact that it is occasionally absent from the placenta. This deficiency is genetically determined and occurs only in the male placenta. In the presence of a sulphatase deficiency the mother has a very low plasma oestriol and urinary oestriol excretion but there is no evidence of increased fetal risk other than the possibility of delay in the onset of labour. It follows that oestriol can hardly be playing a major role in the mother if its absence has so little effect and that, if oestriol has a hormonal function in its own right, it is more likely to be exercised in the fetus than the mother.

Another enzyme system of clinical interest is the aromatising enzymes which convert ring A of the neutral steroid androgens into the aromatic (phenolic) ring which characterises oestrogens. If the fetal circulation is cut off, placental progesterone synthesis continues but maternal oestriol levels decline. It was first suggested that the aromatising system was particularly sensitive to a fall in oxygen concentration and that it was the decline in placental oxygenation, secondary to a decrease in uterine blood flow, which led to a fall in maternal oestriol. The balance of probability has now swung against this supposition; it is more likely that the fall in oestriol is engendered by a decline in the supply of fetal precursors.

The basic substrate for placental oestrogen synthesis is dehydroepiandrosterone, a C19 androgen. Although the main supply of dehydroepiandrosterone comes from the fetus the placenta is equally able to utilise dehydroepiandrosterone of maternal origin. An interesting dynamic placental function test, which has never met with much enthusiasm in clinical circles, is to inject dehydroepiandrosterone or its sulphate into the pregnant woman and observe the subsequent rise of oestradiol. Although several placental enzymes are involved in this transformation it is likely that the limiting factor is 3β-hydroxysteroid dehydrogenase. The dehydroepiandrosterone–oestradiol test is therefore largely a test of placental 3β-dehydroxysteroid dehydrogenase activity. It appears, however, that this enzyme is not easily affected by adverse placental conditions. The test, although of great interest in the study of oestrogen metabolism in pregnancy, has found little clinical application.

References

Curzen P, Southcombe C (1970) The relation between heat-stable alkaline phosphatase in maternal serum and urinary oestrogen output. J Obstet Gynaecol Br Commonwealth 77: 97
Curzen P, Varma R (1971) A comparison of serum heat-stable alkaline phosphatase and urinary oestrogen excretion in the mother as placental function tests. J Obstet Gynaecol Br Commonwealth 78: 686
Elder MG (1971) Serum heat-stable alkaline phosphatase levels and their relation to urinary oestrogen output and fetal and placental weights. J Obstet Gynaecol Br Commonwealth 78: 123
Gottlieb AJ, Sussman HH (1968) Human placental alkaline phosphatase:molecular weight and subunit structure. Biochim Biophys Acta 160: 167
Hagerman DD (1969) The enzymology of the placenta. In: Klopper A, Diczfalusy E (eds) Foetus and placenta. Blackwells, Oxford, pp 413–470
Hensleigh A, Krantz KE (1970) Oxytocinase and placental function. J Obstet Gynecol 107: 1233
Merrett JD, Hunter RJ (1973) Serum heat stable alkaline phosphatase levels in normal and abnormal pregnancies. J Obstet Gynaecol Br Commonwealth 80: 957
Shane JM, Suzuki K (1974) Placental alkaline phosphatase: A review and re-evaluation of its applicability in monitoring fetoplacental function. Obstet Gynecol Survey 29: 97
Tovey JE (1969) Serum oxytocinase. Clin Biochem 2: 289
Watson D, Siddiqui SA, Stafford JEH, Gibbard S, Hewitt V (1973) A comparative study of five laboratory tests for fœto-placental dysfunction in late pregnancy. J Clin Pathol 26: 294

Chapter 5
Steroid Hormones

The steroids are a class of compounds ranging from cholesterol, which has 27 carbon atoms, to testosterone, which has 19. Their common feature is the cyclophenanthrene nucleus: a structure of four conjoined carbon rings, three of which are six membered and one of which is five membered. We shall be concerned with only two sorts of steroid: oestrogens and progestogens.

Oestrogens

The oestrogens have 18 carbon atoms and one ring is aromatic—it has double bonds between alternate carbon atoms. This ring also has a hydroxyl (OH) group on the fourth carbon atom. Such a structure is characteristic of phenols and gives to the oestrogens some chemical properties not shared by other, neutral steroids.

Some 27 oestrogens have been isolated from the urine of pregnant women and their structure determined. We shall consider only two or three oestrogens, production of which have been used as measures of fetal wellbeing. One of these, oestriol, is produced in very large quantities relative to the others in pregnancy. Its measurement has dominated the use of oestrogen assay for the assessment of placental function and we shall concentrate on it, mentioning other oestrogens only in passing.

Most oestrogens produce a yellow colour in sulphuric acid. When this is diluted with water the colour turns pink—the Kober reaction. This Kober colour is fairly specific for oestrogens, and its spectrophotometric measurement has been widely used for the determination of oestrogens, often without attempting to separate the various oestrogens which contribute to the colour. Although such non-specific measurement does violence to the word, total oestrogen assays are in widespread use. Their redeeming feature is that pregnancy urine contains a close correlation between total oestrogen and oestriol; therefore in this chapter the assays will be considered together under the generic title of oestriol.

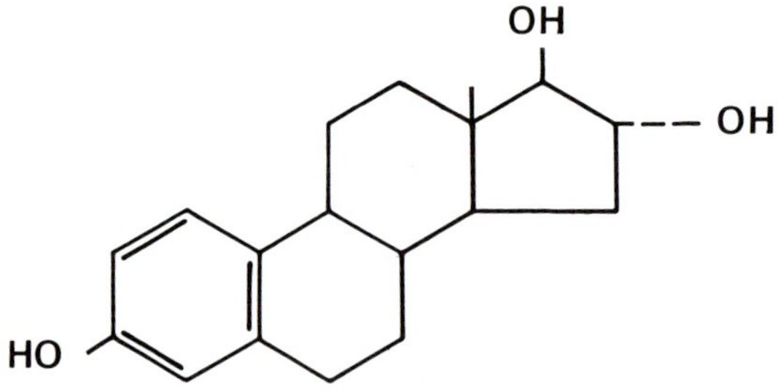

Fig. 5.1. The structure of oestriol.

Oestriol

Isolation and characterisation

Marrian (1930) isolated from the urine of pregnant women a trihydroxy phenol which was later called oestriol (Fig. 5.1). Like other oestrogens it has an aromatic ring A with a hydroxyl at carbon 3, but is distinguished by the substituents on C17 and C16. The two chemical near relatives of oestriol are oestrone and oestradiol. Oestrone has only one hydroxyl group, C3. Oestradiol has two, at C3 and C17. Oestriol has three, at C3, C17 and C16. It is the latter which is of particular interest in the assessment of fetal wellbeing. The fetal liver and to a lesser extent the fetal adrenal are particularly well endowed with the enzyme system which adds the hydroxyl group at C16 of the steroid nucleus. Oestriol in maternal blood and urine relates to the activity of this enzyme in the fetus.

Synthesis

Steroids can be synthesised from simple two-carbon acetate fragments. If steroid synthesising tissues such as testis, adrenal or placenta are incubated with radiolabelled acetate, radioactive steroids are produced. To go from acetate to steroid is a complex process, involving many intermediate compounds. All steroid-producing organs possess the array of enzymes necessary for these steps. At the end of this chain is a familiar steroid which is very widely distributed in the animal and vegetable kingdom. This is cholesterol, with 27 carbon atoms. The process of producing particular steroids such as oestriol from cholesterol starts with the enzymatic removal of carbon atoms. As shown in Fig. 5.2 the first step involves the removal of six carbon atoms in the side chain of cholesterol leaving a 21 carbon steroid—pregnenolone. Pregnenolone is the precursor of all the steroids, the last common point

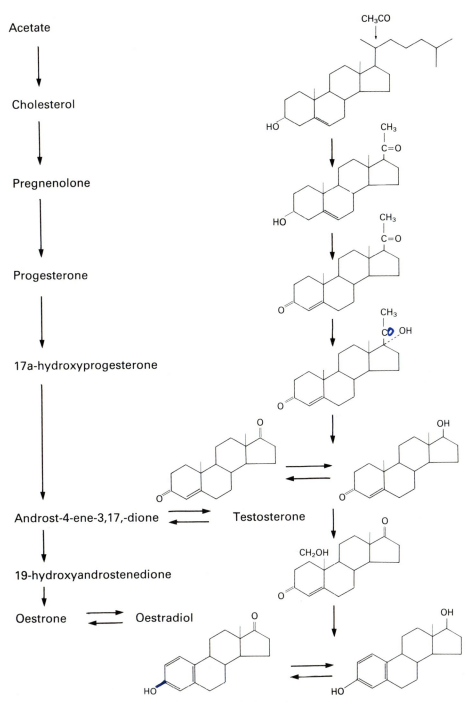

Fig. 5.2. The biosynthesis of oestrogens from cholesterol.

before the pathways diverge to aldosterone, to cortisol, to progesterone, to androgens and to oestrogens. Figure 5.2 shows that in the case of the oestrogens the biosynthetic pathway leads from the C21 steroid pregnenolone to the C19 androgen dehydroepiandrosterone and thence to the C18 oestrogens.

There are large amounts of cholesterol from the dietary intake and from liver synthesis available to all steroid-producing organs. Under physiological circumstances the gonads, the adrenal and the placenta do not start steroid synthesis from acetate fragments but use cholesterol, which is present in such abundance that if all forms of cholesterol were equally useful there would be no question of substrate limitation exerting any control over synthesis. There is good evidence that tissues producing steroid hormones use only the cholesterol that is contained in the low-density lipoprotein fraction of serum (Winkel et al. 1980). Even so the connection between substrate supply and the production of any steroid is at most remote and the critical rate-limiting steps have to be sought further down the chain.

The belief that the placenta is the dominant endocrine gland of pregnancy held sway until the end of the 1950s. Then Diczfalusy put forward the idea of the fetoplacental unit (Diczfalusy 1962). The concept that the fetus itself plays a part in the biosynthesis of steroids (Diczfalusy and Mancuso 1969) has dominated research in this field and is the key to the genesis of oestriol. The demonstration of the fetal role in the formation of oestriol held out the hope that by measuring this steroid, more than any other placental product, we could hold up a mirror to the fetus. In essence, Diczfalusy suggested that neither placenta nor fetus was a complete endocrine entity in itself, but that each held a separate array of enzymes able to carry out particular steps in the synthesis of oestriol. Thus the placenta can convert cholesterol to pregnenolone and further to progesterone, a process which the fetus cannot do to any extent. The first step in converting a C21 steroid like pregnenolone to a C19 androgen consists in the insertion of a hydroxyl group at C17. Neither this, nor the subsequent removal of two carbon atoms to convert C21 pregnenolone to C19 dehydroepiandrosterone, can be done in the placenta. The placenta therefore delivers pregnenolone to the fetal adrenal, which returns dehydroepiandrosterone to the placenta. The placenta is very rich in 3β-hydroxysteroid dehydrogenase, which changes the double bond at C5 in ring B to one at C4 in ring A, and at the same time oxidises the hydroxyl group at C3 to a keto group. This enzyme may well constitute a rate-limiting step in the synthesis of the oestrogens. The activity of 3β-hydroxysteroid dehydrogenase results in the formation of androgens like androstenedione and testosterone, all characterised by the Δ4-3 ketene grouping. Such androgens are the immediate precursors of the oestrogens. The methyl (CH3) group at C19 is removed leaving a C18 steroid in which ring A is aromatised by a placental aromatising enzyme. Although the biosynthesis of the oestrogens requires the molecules to be shuttled back and forth between the fetus and placenta (Diczfalusy's fetoplacental unit) the last step is performed in the placenta and it is from here that the oestrogens are distributed. There is a high concentration of various oestrogens in the fetal circulation and it is generally assumed that placental secretion is bidirectional; into both fetal and maternal circulations. In the case of the protein hormones the secretion is unidirectional into the maternal circulation. It is possible that most of the placental steroid production goes to the fetus and that most of the oestrogens which eventually appear in the maternal circulation do so by transmission from the fetal circulation, having fulfilled their primary function in the fetus. This hypothesis has two important implications. Firstly we should seek the functions of the oestrogens in the fetus as well as in the mother. Secondly maternal oestrogen concentrations will be determined partly by placental transmission; a process which, as we shall see, involves quite a different set of enzymes from those of fetoplacental biosynthesis and therefore introduces the possibility of other rate-limiting steps.

The hydroxyl group at C16 of oestriol is of particular interest to the assessment of fetal wellbeing. This group can be attached to the steroid nucleus at many points in the biosynthetic chain, notably pregnenolone and dehydroepiandrosterone. Although oestrogens such as oestrone and oestradiol can be hydroxylated at C16 (indeed this is the main pathway of oestriol formation in non-pregnant women) it is generally accepted that 16-hydroxy-dehydroepiandrosterone is the main precursor of oestriol in pregnancy. The importance of this finding lies in the fact that the fetal liver is rich in 16-hydroxylating enzymes while the placenta is not. This, as much as any other step in oestriol biosynthesis, accounts for the fetal element in determining oestriol production.

In theory the high concentration of biologically potent androgens and oestrogens in the fetoplacental unit might cause untoward effects in the fetus. However, the bulk of these steroids do not exist in the free, biologically active form, but as sulphates. The true precursor of the oestrogens is not dehydroepiandrosterone but dehydroepiandrosterone sulphate. In turn the main oestriol moiety in the fetal circulation is oestriol sulphate, conjugated in the fetal liver, which is rich in sulphuryl transferase. The placenta, on the other hand, has a high content of sulphatase and placental transmission of oestriol is preceded by hydrolysis of the sulphate. Hence the possibility exists that placental sulphatase may constitute a critical rate-limiting step in determining maternal oestriol concentration. Once hydrolysed, the oestriol is transmitted in the unconjugated form and rapidly reconjugated in the mother, this time mainly as glucosiduronates. A small amount of oestriol glucosiduronate is formed in the fetus and transmitted as such, but by far the major part of the oestriol is transmitted after hydrolysis of the sulphate. Oestriol glucosiduronate is excreted by the kidney by active tubular excretion as well as by glomerular filtration and thus the main form of oestriol in maternal urine is oestriol-16-glucosiduronate.

Metabolism

Only 5%–8% of the total oestriol in the mother's circulation exists as the free steroid; the rest is conjugated and therefore biologically inactive. The concentration of conjugates may bear little relevance to the population of biologically active molecules at the target site and less to the rate of production by the fetoplacental unit. Free oestradiol in the circulation is bound by a specific, characterised protein. An equivalent carrier protein for oestriol has not been identified although it is possible that one exists. Oestrogens exert their action by penetrating the cell membrane and being bound by a protein in the cytoplasm of oestrogen-sensitive cells. If oestriol is bound to a carrier protein only the small unbound fraction can freely enter cells. The concentration of carrier protein may be an important factor in determining how much unconjugated oestriol is free to enter cells as is the case with oestradiol. In terms of biologically available oestriol, even measurements of the unconjugated steroid may be deceptive.

One feature of oestriol metabolism makes measurements of this steroid attractive vis à vis other oestrogens. Oestrone differs from oestradiol only in having a keto group at C17 in place of a hydroxyl group, i.e. by one hydrogen atom. The transhydrogenation system which can convert one into the other is widely distributed and the concentration of oestrone or oestradiol will be determined by the equilibrium between the two. Oestriol, on the other hand, is an end product. Its concentration is not affected by conversion to other oestrogens.

Compartmental distribution

Steroids are distributed through all body compartments including the interstitial fluid, the intracellular space and the body fat. They flow in and out of these compartments and between the mother and the fetoplacental unit with greater or lesser freedom. It follows that fetoplacental oestriol production is not the sole source of inflow. Indeed when fetoplacental production is sharply reduced, inflow from other maternal compartments dampens the fall in plasma oestriol concentration. Around one-third to one-half of the fetoplacental steroid load in the maternal circulation is diverted to the bile (Adlercreutz 1974) and clearly this has a profound effect on plasma oestriol levels and even on the urinary excretion. The main biliary form of oestriol is oestriol-3-sulphate-16-glucosiduronate (Levitz and Katz 1968), which is hydrolysed in the gut. It is then reconjugated in the gut wall as oestriol-3-glucosiduronate and reabsorbed into the maternal circulation.

If by measurements on maternal blood or urine, one wishes to gain information on fetoplacental production, it is wise to avoid those forms of the steroid most involved in the enterohepatic circulation. In the maternal plasma the forms of choice for assay would be either unconjugated oestriol or oestriol-3-sulphate. The kidney has the capacity to metabolise unconjugated oestriol to oestriol glucosiduronates and excrete the latter in urine (Kirdani et al. 1972). It would appear that the urinary form of oestriol most directly related to fetoplacental production is oestriol-16-glucosiduronate.

Biological function

Oestrogens are concerned with growth, with cellular proliferation in oestrogen-sensitive organs. Oestrogens, in particular oestradiol, deliver at the genome in the nucleus of the cells of the endometrium, the myometrium and the breast, a message which leads to fresh protein synthesis. But their effects go well beyond cell proliferation and extend to many metabolic aspects such as vascular permeability and fluid balance. The enlargement of intravascular volume and the increase in total body water, which are such a marked feature of pregnancy, are as much an oestrogen effect as the growth of the uterus and the breasts. Indeed many of the maternal adaptations to pregnancy are mediated by oestrogens. It is as though oestrogens were a tool with which the fetus reaches into the mother, resetting her metabolic controls to meet the needs of pregnancy.

Some of the features of oestriol production during pregnancy are difficult to reconcile with any theories concerning the function of this steroid. Why should it rise steadily throughout pregnancy, reaching levels more than a thousand times higher than at the beginning? What activity in pregnancy needs such a steady increase? It may be that new processes connected with say, cervical distensibility or with myometrial contractility are set in train as critical levels are reached. But oestrogen levels vary so greatly from one normal woman to another at the same stage of gestation, that it is difficult to believe that there are any critical levels.

The mother is not necessarily the prime target of the oestrogens produced in pregnancy; it could be the fetus. There is indeed a fairly close connection between fetal size and oestriol levels, although this is more likely *post hoc* than *propter hoc*. The neuroendocrine development of the fetus, and perhaps other aspects of sexual differentiation, are under oestrogen influence.

The most unhappy feature of our understanding of the biological function of oestrogens in pregnancy is that we are unable to locate any activity unique to oestriol, as opposed to other oestrogens. Is there anything this molecule will do that none of the others can do? There is no way of controverting the suggestion that oestriol is metabolic garbage, a convenient way of getting rid of oestrogens. Then why so much trouble to make so much of that particular oestrogen by a pathway not involving other oestrogens? The question is teleological but legitimate. Until we answer it we are well short of knowing how best to use oestriol assays.

Control of production

Small fetuses produce less oestriol than do larger ones of the same gestational age. It might therefore be assumed that control of oestriol production resides in the fetus. But this is altogether too simple. For one thing, fetal and placental weight are related and it might well be that both fetal size and oestriol production are dependent on the placenta. Also some fetuses are growth retarded and possibly fetal size and oestriol production are independent and secondary consequences of a primary pathology. On the other hand various lines of experiment have identified the activity of certain enzyme systems as rate-limiting steps. In the placenta the prime candidates are 3β-hydroxysteroid dehydrogenase and placental aromatase. In the fetus the critical steps are C16 hydroxylation and the removal of the side chain at C21.

In rare instances, such as sulphatase deficiency, it is possible to identify a single rate-limiting step, but more often one gains the impression that substrate supply from the fetal adrenal, more than anything else, determines how much oestriol is being made. In the last resort, whatever controls the fetal adrenal also controls oestriol biosynthesis. How far fetal adrenals are under control of the fetal pituitary is difficult to say. At one time it was thought that chorionic gonadotrophin was the determining factor in the production of dehydroepiandrosterone, but there is no direct connection between hCG on the one hand and dehydroepiandrosterone and oestriol on the other.

It is likely that changes in the control of oestriol production occur during the course of gestation. Klopper and Billewicz (1963) speculated that the surge of oestriol production which starts at 34 weeks gestation was a specifically fetal process, a new factor in oestriol biogenesis engendered in late pregnancy.

In one sense our understanding of the control of oestriol production is sadly lacking. Oestrogen production by the gonads is regulated by a feedback mechanism of the oestrogens themselves on the pituitary. There is no evidence of any such mechanism in the control of oestriol production by the fetoplacental unit. There appears to be no means by which the fetoplacental unit can sense when it is producing too little, too much or just enough oestriol. The system appears to be running free. This is a great weakness in the use of oestriol assays: we do not know what process we are measuring.

Methods of measurement

In late pregnancy a 24-h urine specimen contains 20–30 mg oestriol. One millilitre contains many micrograms and measurement is well within the power of spectrophotometry when that amount of oestriol is converted by the Kober reaction (Kober 1931). The problem is that the Kober reaction is not specific to oestriol; it can be produced by any oestrogen and very similar colours are produced by other substances in urine. In addition the generation of the colour is influenced by many impurities which may be present in the final reaction. Urinary oestriol assays were therefore always beset by the difficulties of first extracting the steroid from urine and then purifying it. This problem was solved in the technique evolved by Brown (1955) but this method was laborious and ill adapted for handling the many assays generated by the application of urinary oestriol determinations as a means of assessing fetal state. Less specific short-cut methods, one evolved by Brown himself (Brown and Coyle 1963), came into use and made possible many thousands of assays. However, such assays are an uneasy compromise between convenience and specificity. In essence they depend on hydrolysis of the oestriol conjugates, extraction of the free steroid, a greater or lesser degree of purification of the extract, production of a Kober colour and reading this by spectrophotometry of fluorimetry. Most so-called oestriol assays are an outrage on the chemical designation, but serve well in obstetric practice. The ability to do many assays within a day has more than compensated for the fact that the answers bore only a somewhat haphazard relevance to the real oestriol content of the urine.

Some claims were advanced for plasma oestriol assays using established urinary techniques, but practical plasma assays had to await the appearance of RIA in the late 1960s. This transformed the scene, making it possible to measure picograms of oestriol with reasonable specificity and accuracy. Oestriol, like other steroids, is not immunogenic on its own and antibodies could only be produced by conjugating it with a foreign protein. When, for example, oestriol antibodies are to be produced in a rabbit, the steroid is commonly conjugated to bovine serum albumin. The first antisera were produced by attaching the steroid to the protein at some convenient site on the steroid molecule, such as the phenolic hydroxyl on C3. This tended to obscure characteristic features of the structure of the molecule from the antibody-forming mechanism and, as a result, the antisera could not distinguish between, say, oestriol and oestradiol. The second generation of antisera was more sophisticated. The attachment to the protein was made at a point in the steroid nucleus which left the characteristic substituents exposed. In the case of oestriol this commonly involved making the connection at C6. Such antisera are able to discriminate between molecules to a fine degree. As regards oestriol they can discriminate between oestriol and epioestriol, i.e. they can read the orientation of the hydroxyl group at C16.

What remains to be done on the methodology of plasma oestriol assay is cosmetic, not revolutionary. Extraction of the free steroid from the plasma before estimation is still necessary for most methods but some claims are being advanced for antisera robust enough to be successfully used on untreated plasma or serum. RIAs are difficult to automate for large-scale turnover, and require sophisticated, expensive apparatus. Enzyme immunoassays and fluoroimmunoassays are attractive in these respects and may well replace RIAs.

Blood versus urine

The relative merits of assays done on serum or plasma have been hotly debated. There is so much to be said on either side that the argument cannot be resolved. It is worthwhile rehearsing some of the arguments so that the reader may draw conclusions in terms of his own circumstances.

The choice between blood and urine depends on the objective of the oestriol assay. If one wishes to gain insight into how much oestriol is available to the target organ, there is little doubt about the superiority of plasma assays. But the purpose of oestriol assays in studies of placental function is to determine the rate of production of the steroid by the fetoplacental unit. With that in mind, the advantage may lie with urinary assay; particularly when one remembers that urinary assays provide a summary of the production rate over the previous 24 h, while a plasma concentration figure applies to only a moment in time—that moment when the blood was drawn.

Blood is a turbulent pool with many streams of oestriol flowing in and out of it. We have already pointed out some of the objections to the assumption that maternal plasma concentration necessarily reflects the rate of production by the fetoplacental unit. Even when the fetoplacental input is the determining factor of plasma oestriol concentration, the value of any concentration figure depends upon an even rate of inflow. Oestriol has a short residence time in the circulation and may fluctuate in response to short-term variations of input which have no physiological significance. If, as has been argued elsewhere, uterine blood flow is an important factor in determining the concentration of a hormone in the peripheral circulation of the mother, changes in blood flow may cause marked changes in plasma concentration without necessarily representing any change in fetoplacental production. These minute-to-minute variations in plasma oestriol concentration have led some investigators to regard single estimations as unrepresentative, and to recommend that oestriol assays should be the average of repeated samples (Buster et al. 1978).

Urine samples are bulky to store and transport, offensive to handle, and tedious and difficult to collect. These convenience factors would not be important if urinary assays gave information inherently more useful than plasma assays. They bulk large if the two are anywhere near comparable. The fact that very few units, having started plasma assays, have ever gone back to urinary assays, suggests that the plasma concentration figure gives information comparable with that from urinary assays.

Comparisons between blood and urine should not be pursued too far. Clinicians are apt to regard plasma assays as a sophisticated form of urinary measurement. Nothing could be further from the truth. The difference between urinary and plasma assays has been examined in detail elsewhere (Klopper 1976a) and will not be pursued here. Suffice it to say they are related but different concepts. To say one is a truer reflection of fetal wellbeing than the other is false: each is a mirror held up to a different aspect of the truth, and each reflection is a distortion.

Variability

It is intended to include under the single heading of variability two concepts (time and person) and two fluids (blood and urine). The variability differences between blood and urine are trivial and will for the most part be ignored. Variability from time to time and from person to person are different concepts and require separate consideration (Klopper 1976b).

Time-to-time variability. Plasma oestriol can vary with time in numerous ways: there may be spurts of input from minute to minute from the fetoplacental unit, presumably reflecting changes in uterine blood flow. There may be slow diurnal changes reflecting timing mechanisms in the fetal adrenal. Maternal events such as exercise, posture or eating a meal may affect oestriol levels. None of these affect 24-h urinary excretion, which of itself contains all the events of the previous 24 h. The fact that day-to-day variability in plasma oestriol concentration or in 24 h urinary excretion is much the same indicates that none of these sources of variability have much effect on plasma oestriol. There is controversy as to whether plasma oestriol levels show consistent changes during the day (i.e. a rhythm). However, these changes are small and inconsistent, and can be easily avoided by drawing blood at the same time each day; an activity which accords well with the proclivity of most wards for a settled, regular routine. Physiological events such as exercise have no consistent predictable effect on plasma oestriol concentration (Klopper et al. 1974). In the end, the change from day to day in a patient is the critical variant in clinical practice. Of course, daily measurements contain an element of variation due to the measurements themselves. This is not inconsiderable, as for most RIA techniques the interassay coefficient of variation is around 10%. When one considers that the overall day-to-day coefficient of variation in plasma oestriol is 14% it is remarkable how steady the plasma levels really are (Klopper et al. 1974). Surprisingly, the day-to-day urinary excretion is slightly more variable, 18% (Klopper et al. 1969). There is little to choose between urine and blood or between one steroid and another in terms of variability from time to time.

Person-to-person variability. The high variability in the plasma concentration or the urinary excretion of oestriol from one person to another is one of the main stumbling blocks in the use of oestriol assays to assess placental function. The coefficient of variation in a large group of normal women all at the same stage of gestation was 32% (Klopper et al. 1974). Likely factors such as maternal weight, age or parity have no consistent effect and cannot be allowed for. Like other parameters considered in this book, the distribution of normal values is skewed; that is, there are more observations below than above the arithmetic mean, which is drawn up by a few wildly high values. This odd phenomenon is difficult to explain but its effects as far as the clinical application of hormone assays is concerned can be reduced by a simple mathematical trick. This is to do a logarithmic or square root transform of the values. This does not affect the normal range in the sense of standard deviations about the mean but it does raise the value of the lower limit, while at the same time increasing the upper limit, and provides a better approximation to the actual spread of values.

Normal range during pregnancy. Until recently normal ranges were calculated in terms of standard deviation about the mean at each stage of gestation. This value has a 30% or greater coefficient of variation at each stage of gestation. The 95% confidence limits are therefore more than 60% above and below the mean, and this wide range will inevitably include most of the clinically abnormal patients. Probably the best way to represent the normal range is by non-parametric statistics such as the median and centiles. Although this does nothing to reduce the problem of the wide range, it gives the observer the satisfaction of knowing what percentage of normals would be included in a particular value.

The most puzzling and disappointing feature of the wide normal range is that we cannot account for it. The differences in oestriol concentration from one woman to another cannot be explained by any one feature such as maternal size, age, parity, placental weight or any other variable. Fetal size has only an indirect connection with oestriol production and is not necessarily causal.

The mean normal curve. Some parameters, e.g. hPL, are clearly reflections of the functional mass of the trophoblast. Placental growth slows up in the last few weeks of pregnancy and so does the increase in such parameters. However, plasma or urinary oestriol continue to rise right up to term. This is helpful as it may make it easier to detect subtle changes in oestriol levels. Fetal growth retardation in particular does not always lead to an overt fall in oestriol in late pregnancy but may manifest itself by a failure of the continuous rise in serial measurements. Such a phenomenon may be difficult to detect when one compares one day's results with those of the previous day, but becomes more obvious if a running mean is constructed.

In early pregnancy growth rates in terms of proportionate increase are high and the relative increase in oestriol is steep. If the mean values are expressed in logarithmic terms one gets a straight line. Such log plots are difficult to use in terms of the day-to-day arithmetic values and tend to conceal as much as they reveal. The complexity of the mean oestriol curve is shown in Figure 5.3, with a steep initial rise, a flattening in mid-pregnancy and a further rise up to term in late pregnancy.

Clinical applications—early pregnancy

There are few studies on oestriol changes in early pregnancy. Most attention has focussed on those hormones presumed to be concerned with the maintenance of pregnancy, notably chorionic gonadotrophin and progesterone. As a cause of spontaneous abortion primary hormonal failure is not important. Hormone levels are more likely to reflect established fetoplacental damage than to be causally involved and the purpose of hormone assays lies more in prognosis than in indicating the need for specific endocrine therapy. There are two situations in which such hormone assays may serve a useful purpose. One is recurrent abortion and the other is threatened abortion. When a woman has a history of repeated early pregnancy loss it is difficult to forecast the outcome of a current pregnancy. It is often not appreciated that recurrent abortion may have its genesis early in the pregnancy—at implantation or soon after. Hormone assays at 10 or 12 weeks' gestation come much too late after the event. Indeed some of the most successful studies have preceded the pregnancy in the proliferative phase before ovulation. Here, of course, one is studying the hormone production of the ovary, not the placenta. As oestradiol, not oestriol, is the oestrogen produced by the follicle it is likely that oestradiol assays will give the most reliable indication of the functional state of the Graafian follicle from which the pregnancy arose.

After the trophoblast has taken over endocrine function from the ovary (at 7–8 weeks), it is generally thought that progesterone rather than oestriol is the most reliable indicator. There is no strong reason why this should be so and experimental observations do not support it. The oestriol:oestradiol ratio shifts in favour of oestriol very early in pregnancy and it is evident that the

Oestriol

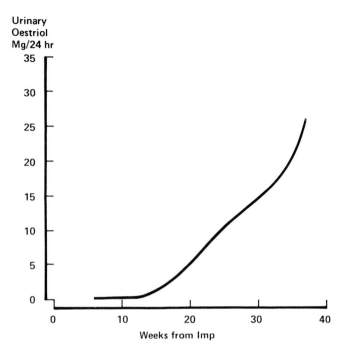

Fig. 5.3. The shape of the mean oestriol excretion curve during pregnancy.

fetoplacental pattern of oestrogen production, as contrasted with ovarian, is biased towards oestriol. Conceptual failure is as likely to be fetoplacental as purely placental in origin and in terms of what has already been said about the fetal role in the genesis of oestriol, it is not surprising that this steroid appears to be most closely tuned to the fetal state. In a study of recurrent abortion Klopper and MacNaughton (1965) found the fall of urinary oestriol occurred earlier and was more consistent than the fall in pregnanediol in those patients who went on to abort. In threatened abortion too, oestriol assays are more reliable than measurements of progesterone or urinary pregnanediol, although it must be admitted that a substantial fall in steroid production seldom precedes clinical diagnosis in a useful manner.

Because the fetus is absent in hydatidiform mole and choriocarcinoma it was thought that these conditions would be characterised by very low oestriol levels. This is true to some extent but not sufficiently so to be useful, and ultrasonic examination and chorionic gonadotrophin assays provide more secure means of diagnosis.

Clinical applications—late pregnancy

It is not reasonable to assume that all complications of late pregnancy will affect oestriol production equally or indeed affect it at all. The disease states need to be strictly categorised and the oestriol levels in each examined separately.

Perhaps the commonest condition in which obstetricians are likely to turn to hormone assays is retarded intrauterine fetal growth—the light-for-dates baby. There is a correlation between plasma or urinary oestriol and fetal weight, and generally speaking oestriol is low when fetal weight is low. The problem is that fetal growth retardation is the outcome of a variety of causes; each of which might operate differently on oestriol production. Factors such as maternal hypertension, malnutrition or fetal deformity are all different diseases, although they may all result in the common end point of a growth-retarded baby. Almost all authors agree that fetal growth retardation is associated with low oestriol production but few have considered the oestriol levels in terms of other factors bearing on fetal weight, such as maternal weight gain and blood pressure. Such a categorisation was attempted by Masson (1973). He found that the changes in plasma oestriol were most marked when the fetal growth retardation was accompanied by maternal hypertension. The pattern of oestriol in such women was that the oestriol rise after 30 weeks was very slight and the levels tended to fall after 37 weeks. He concluded that, because of the overlap between normal and growth-retarded oestriol values, the measurements were not good as a means of diagnosis but that serial assays were useful in clinical control.

Pre-eclamptic toxaemia is a diverse disease and the accompanying changes in oestriol production may vary widely. Although not amenable to strict proof, it is likely that the origin of toxaemia lies in the placenta rather than in the fetus. It is probable that changes in plasma or urinary oestriol in toxaemia reflect placental rather than fetal events. Thus, the fall in oestriol production commonly found in toxaemia is most likely the outcome of placental damage such as infarction rather than directly a measure of fetal vitality.

Pre-eclamptic toxaemia, by definition, is diagnosed with a sphygmomanometer and by urinary protein measurement. Therefore measurement of oestriol is not diagnostic in pre-eclampsia, although some evidence suggests that the fall in oestriol is related to the severity of the disease. The application of oestriol assays lies in the possibility of predicting the course of the disease or the outcome as far as the fetus is concerned; in other words, as one additional factor in deciding when to effect delivery, or the likely condition of the fetus at delivery.

Diabetic pregnancy presents even more diverse aspects. Sometimes one is dealing with a large baby and a proportionately large placenta. On other occasions the pregnancy manifests toxaemia and results in the delivery of a growth-retarded baby with an undergrown, infarcted placenta. Not surprisingly the oestriol levels may differ widely. Oestriol measurements in diabetic pregnancy have always been viewed with more enthusiasm in the United States than in Britain. In many American centres oestriol assays are a very important component of clinical management. A critical appraisal of the results does not encourage this view.

One criterion of reproductive performance is simply whether a pregnancy produces a live or a dead fetus. When a baby dies in utero, it is not difficult to determine this fact, and oestriol assays are hardly necessary. Their use is in assessing in advance the risk of intrauterine death. Oestriol changes before intrauterine death are controlled by two factors—the time before death and the cause for the fetal demise. When fetal death is sudden, due to retroplacental haemorrhage, the oestriol levels may be normal up to a few minutes before the event. When a hypertensive woman has a slow intrauterine death of a growth retarded fetus, the fact may be signalled a week or more in advance by falling oestriol.

It is as well to state the worst case. The work of Klopper and Stephenson (1966) made it clear that in Rh-incompatible pregnancy, oestriol levels gave no indication as to whether the fetus was severely affected or not at all. Many instances have been recorded where maternal plasma or urinary oestriol were well within normal limits when the fetus was moribund.

Other oestrogens

Although oestriol assays have long dominated the field in the assessment of placental function, from time to time other oestrogens have been examined. Oestrone and oestradiol are interconvertible and it matters little which one of the two is selected. Oestradiol rises steeply during pregnancy and there is little doubt that its levels bear some relation to placental function. There is no good reason to suppose that this relationship is any closer than that of oestriol. By virtue of the fact that oestradiol lacks the essentially fetal step of 16-hydroxylation in its biosynthesis it is likely to be a less accurate reflection of the fetal state than oestriol.

Oestetrol has enjoyed a brief vogue. It is presumed to be made predominantly in the fetus from oestradiol (Gurpide et al. 1966), and is found in measurable amounts only during pregnancy. The initial promise of these measurements has not been borne out by experience and plasma oestetrol measurements are now seldom used.

The conversion of DHAS to oestradiol held great promise as a dynamic test of placental function. At first the metabolic clearance rate of radiolabelled DHA was used (Gant et al. 1974) but measuring the rise of oestradiol produced by the intravenous injection of 50 mg DHAS proved more convenient and acceptable to hospital ethical committees. Unfortunately this interesting dynamic test has also not proved to be clinically reliable. On occasion normal conversions have been recorded when the fetus was moribund.

Progestogens

Although several C21 steroids related to progesterone increase during pregnancy, the only substantial body of evidence regarding the measurement of progestogens in pregnancy applies to progesterone itself, and measurements of this steroid have proved of little value in the measurement of placental function. Although they may have a modest place in the management of threatened and recurrent abortion they are, in this context, as much measures of ovarian as of placental function. It is disappointing and a little surprising that plasma progesterone should bear so little relevance to the outcome of the pregnancy. It is the sole end point of a short, entirely placental pathway. It has a brief half-life, is biologically active, and is present in very high concentration as compared to other steroids. Its high variability from time to time is a disadvantage but the main drawback is that the placenta retains its capacity to synthesise progesterone unimpaired when other placental functions are seriously impaired. Measurements of the main progesterone metabolite in urine, pregnanediol, give less variable results, but do not yield better information than oestriol assays and have been largely replaced by the latter.

References

Adlercreute, H (1974) Hepatic metabolism of oestrogens in health and disease. N Engl J Med 240: 1081
Brown JB (1955) A chemical method for the determination of oestriol, oestrone and oestradiol in urine. Biochem J 60: 185
Brown JB, Coyle M (1963) Urinary excretion of oestriol during pregnancy. A shortened procedure. J Obstet Gynaecol Br Commonwealth 70: 219
Buster JE, Meis PJ, Hobel CJ, Marshall JR (1978) Subhourly variability of circulating third trimester maternal steroid concentrations as a source of sampling error. J Clin Endocrinol Metab 46: 907–910
Diczfalusy E (1962) The endocrinology of the fetus. Acta Obstet Gynecol Scand 41 [Suppl 1] 45–85
Diczfalusy E, Mancuso S (1969) Oestrogen metabolism in pregnancy. In: Klopper A, Diczfalusy E (eds) Foetus and placenta. Blackwells, Oxford, pp 191–148
Gant N, Hutchinson H, Siiteri P, MacDonald P (1971) Study of the metabolic clearance rate of dehydroisoandrosterone sulfate in pregnancy. Am J Obstet Gynecol 111: 555
Gurpide E, Schwers J, Welch M, Van de Wiele R, Lieberman S (1966 Fetal and maternal metabolism of estradiol during pregnancy. J Clin Endocrinol Metab 26: 1355
Halbert SP, Lin T-M (1979) Pregnancy-associated plasma proteins: PAPP-A and PAPP-B In: Klopper A, Chard T (eds) Placental proteins. Springer-Verlag, Berlin, Heidelberg, New York, pp 89–103
Kirdani RY, Sampson D, Murphy GP, Sandberg AA (1972) Studies on phenolic steroids in human subjects. J Clin Endocrinol Metab 34: 546
Klopper A (1976a) Criteria for the selection of steroid assays in the assessment of fetoplacental function. In: Klopper A (ed) Plasma hormone assays in the evaluation of fetal wellbeing. Churchill Livingstone, Edinburgh, pp 20–35
Klopper A (1976b) The choice between assays on blood or on urine. In: Loraine JH, Bell ET (eds) Hormone assays and their clinical application. Churchill Livingstone, Edinburgh, pp 74–86
Klopper A, Billewicz Z (1963) Urinary excretion of oestriol and pregnanediol during pregnancy. J Obstet Gynaecol Br Commonwealth 70: 1024
Klopper A, MacNaughton M (1965) Hormones in recurrent abortion. J Obstet Gynaecol Br Commonwealth 77: 102
Klopper A, Stephenson R (1966) The excretion of pregnanediol and of oestriol in pregnancy complicated by Rh immunisation. J Obstet Gynaecol Br Commonwealth 73: 982
Klopper A, Wilson G, Cooke I (1969) Variability of urinary steroid excretion. J Endocrinol 43: 295

Klopper A, Wilson G, Masson G (1974) The variability of plasma hormone levels in late pregnancy. In: Scholler R (ed) Hormonal investigations in human pregnancy. Sepe, Paris, pp 77–86

Kober S (1931) Eine kolorimetrische Bestimmung des Brunshormons (Menformon). Biochem J 239: 209

Levitz M, Katz J (1968) Enterohepatic metabolism of estriol-3-sulphate-16-glucosiduronate in women. J Clin Endocrinol Metab 28: 862

Marrian GF (1930) The chemistry of oestrin. Biochem J 24: 1021

Masson GM (1973) Plasma oestriol in retarded fetal growth. J Obstet Gynaecol Br Commonwealth 80: 206

Winkel CA, MacDonald PC, Simpson ER (1980) The role of maternal circulating low density lipoprotein in regulating placental progesterone biosynthesis. In: Klopper A, Genazzani A, Crosignani P (eds) The human placenta—hormones and proteins. Academic Press, London, pp 401–406

Chapter 6
Placental Protein Hormones (hCG and hPL)

The human placenta secretes a range of protein and small peptide hormones. The latter, which include corticotrophin (ACTH) and releasing factors, are only of academic interest and will not be discussed here. The larger protein hormones [human placental lactogen (hPL); human chorionic gonadotrophin (hCG)] are the subjects of this chapter. Both are widely used in routine clinical practice, but for very different applications. Thus, hPL is a classic 'placental function test' in the sense of ascertaining fetal wellbeing in late pregnancy, whereas hCG is primarily employed as a 'pregnancy test' or for the monitoring of trophoblastic tumours. However, the applications overlap to the extent that both have been used for the monitoring of abnormalities of early pregnancy, in particular threatened abortion.

Discovery

The presence of material with gonadotrophic activity in the urine from pregnant women was first described by Aschheim and Zondek in 1927. The basic observation and the placental origin of the hormone was subsequently confirmed by many other workers. The presence of a placental lactogenic factor was postulated by Ehrhardt in 1936, but a clear definition of this material was not available until the early 1960s (Ito and Higashi 1961; Josimovich and MacLaren 1962).

Chemistry

Chorionic gonadotrophin (hCG) is a glycoprotein with close structural similarities to pituitary luteinising hormone (LH), follicle-stimulating hormone (FSH) and thyroid stimulating hormone (TSH). It consists of two protein chains referred to as the α- and β-subunits. The chains are joined by non-covalent bonds and thus can be separated by relatively mild dissociating conditions. Both subunits have sidechains of carbohydrate residues, principally sialic acid, which constitute some 12% of the molecule on a weight basis. The α-subunit has 92 amino acid residues and is virtually identical with the α-subunits of LH, FSH and TSH. The β-subunit has 145 amino acid residues. Thirty of these, at the carboxy-terminus of the molecule, are unique to hCG.

The remaining 115 residues are very similar to the 115 residues of the β-subunit of LH; 80% of the sequence is identical. The molecular weights of the α-subunit, β-subunit and the whole molecule are 14,930, 23,470 and 38,400 respectively.

Placental lactogen (hPL) is a protein with close similarities to pituitary prolactin and growth hormone. In consists of a single chain of 191 amino acids without carbohydrate residues. There are two intra-chain disulphide (-S-S-) links. The molecular weight is 21,600.

Synthesis

In common with other products of the placenta both hCG and hPL are synthesised exclusively by the trophoblast. In late pregnancy the syncytiotrophoblast is the principal site, though in early pregnancy there is some evidence for synthesis of hCG by the cytotrophoblast. This observation is in accord with the fact that the cytotrophoblast is much more prominent in early pregnancy at the time when hCG secretion reaches a peak.

Within the trophoblast cell the synthesis of the α- and β-subunits of hCG is independent, i.e. there are quite separate messenger RNAs. The two subunits combine in the cell prior to release as intact hCG, and for this reason only small quantities of the free subunits are secreted into the circulation. The production of β-subunit appears to be the rate-limiting factor; the trophoblast can synthesise much greater quantities of α-subunit than β-subunit, but combination of the two is essential for release from the cell.

The synthesis of hPL is simpler than that of hCG since it involves a single messenger RNA producing a single protein. However, in common with many other proteins hPL is initially synthesised in the form of a slightly larger molecule, having an additional 20 amino acids at the NH_2-terminus. This extra sequence is removed as part of the process of secretion (Chard 1981).

Metabolism

Both hCG and hPL are metabolised by the liver and kidneys; in both cases only a small fraction of the total is excreted in the urine. The half-life ($t_{1/2}$: 5–10 h) of hCG in the circulation, estimated from serial samples following delivery of the placenta, shows an initial phase ($t_{1/2}$: 5–10 h) followed by a phase of slower decline ($t_{1/2}$: 30–50 h). Placental lactogen shows a similar pattern of a rapid followed by a slower fall; in the initial rapid phase the half-life is 15–20 min.

Biological functions

A wide range of functions have been proposed for hCG and hPL and are listed in Table 6.1. As noted elsewhere it is very easy to confuse a 'function' (i.e. the role of the hormone in normal physiology) with an 'effect' (i.e. the action of the hormone in an experimental system). The evidence that any of the putative functions shown in Table 6.1 have physiological reality is at best thin. This point is further emphasised by the fact that certain rare pregnancies associated with an almost total and specific deficiency of hPL are in all other respects normal (Nielsen et al. 1979). The argument is anyway academic because the clinical application of hCG and hPL measurements makes no assumptions whatsoever about the biological role of these materials; they are simply used as overall markers of trophoblast activity.

Control mechanisms

hCG concentration in blood rises very steeply in early pregnancy, reaches a peak around 12 weeks and then declines almost as precipitously, to run at about 10% of the peak value for the rest of the pregnancy. hPL concentrations during pregnancy show the familiar sigmoid curve, reminiscent of placental growth. It is unlikely that the same or similar factors can operate to produce both curves. It is reasonable to suppose that in early pregnancy some factor stimulates trophoblastic hCG synthesis. Later in pregnancy this factor either declines or is replaced by another which positively reduces hCG production. No reasonable hypothesis as to what such factors might be has been put forward. Even in culture experiments it is very difficult to manipu-

Table 6.1. Suggested biological functions of hCG and hPL[a]

	Function
hCG	hPL
Maintenance of corpus luteum and steroid production by the corpus luteum (luteotrophic activity)	Growth-promoting activity
	Mammotrophic/lactogenic activity
	Luteotrophic activity
Stimulation of placental progesterone production	Erythropoietic activity
	Mobilisation of free fatty acids
Stimulation of fetal adrenal and production of DHEA	'Anti-insulin' effect on carbohydrate metabolism
Stimulation of fetal gonads, in particular production of testosterone by the testis	Anabolic effect on nitrogen metabolism
Inhibition of maternal-fetal graft rejection	Inhibition of fibrinolysis
	Inhibition of maternal-fetal graft rejection

[a] A very full account is available in Gaspard (1980).

late hCG production in vitro. There is some evidence that cyclic adenosine monophosphate or luteinising hormone-releasing factor will stimulate hCG production in placental explants, but it is difficult to tie this up with control in vivo.

hPL fits much better the model of control by mass of functioning trophoblast, i.e. the protein is being produced at a steady rate per unit of tissue, without any feedback control (Chard 1981). Even here investigators are not agreed on the critical fact of hPL levels being related to placental mass. Some have found this to be the case (Seppälä and Ruoslahti 1970); others have failed to find a relationship between serum hPL and placental weight (Samaan et al. 1971). For the time being the clinical application of hPL assays must rest on the unsatisfactory basis of empirical observations without understanding of the control mechanism.

Measurement[1]

From the time of its discovery in 1927 hCG has been widely used as the standard pregnancy test. Up to the mid 1960s the measurement was by biological assay: injection of urine into frogs, toads, rabbits, rats or mice. This has now been entirely replaced by immunological techniques, the commonest of which involve particle agglutination in tubes or on slides. However, such methods are largely qualitative; they give a yes or no answer to the presence of an early pregnancy. To determine the wellbeing of a pregnancy requires a quantitative test yielding a number which can then be compared with a normal range. The only techniques which can achieve this are RIA or radioreceptor assays.

RIAs for hCG are of two types: those using antibodies to the whole molecule, and those in which the antibodies are directed to the β-subunit of the molecule. Assays of intact hCG are very liable to cross-react with pituitary LH (because of the common α-subunit and the common sections of the β-subunit; see above). Assays directed to the β-subunit alone are considerably more specific and are the method of choice at the present time. It should be emphasised that most so-called β-subunit assays in fact measure intact hCG in urine or blood (which is what is intended), and not free subunits only. Many good commercial kits are available for hCG β-subunit measurement.

The radioreceptor assay (Saxena et al. 1974) is similar in principle to an RIA but uses a naturally occurring receptor from the corpus luteum in place of antibody. This technique has enjoyed some popularity in the USA though in fact it is rather less specific than the β-subunit RIA.

Clinical measurements of hPL in maternal blood are mostly carried out by RIA. There are no problems of specificity: despite the close chemical relationship to growth hormone and prolactin, cross-reactions of antisera are less

---

[1] Accounts of assay methods for hCG and hPL are given in Bagshawe et al. (1979); Chard (1979).

than 1%. Good commercial kits are available[2] and the ease, speed and precision of measurement go some way to explaining the present popularity of this test, especially in Europe.

Time-to-time variation

As emphasised earlier, the time-to-time variation of fetoplacental products in maternal blood may be a very important criterion for choice of a test. Thus, if the variation is very large, interpretation of the test is correspondingly difficult.

There is virtually no information on the time-to-time variation of hCG levels (surprisingly, in view of the very important application in monitoring therapy of trophoblastic tumours). By contrast, hPL has been studied in great detail and has yielded the following conclusions: (1) there is time-to-time variation whether studied over a period of minutes, hours or days; (2) the variation is entirely random and bears no relationship to normal physiological events or to a 24-h cycle (in other words, it is a variation, not a rhythm); and (3) the overall variation is of the order of 5%—10% (Pavlou et al. 1972). In practical terms this indicates that variation of hPL levels is at, or about, the minimum for any placental function test, and that the timing of samples is unimportant.

Normal range

The normal ranges of hCG and hPL follow the skewed distributions described in Chap. 3. An example of a published range for hPL is shown in Fig. 6.1. As with other placental function tests it should be noted that such ranges are not definitive as it is incumbent on all users of such tests to establish their own values. 'Users' in this context will include any laboratory supplying a test based on their own in-house materials, or any commercial manufacturer providing materials in the form of a kit.

Clinical applications of measurement

hCG in early pregnancy

The largest application of hCG measurement is as a qualitative test for the presence of an early pregnancy. The next largest use is quantitative measurement for monitoring therapy of trophoblast tumours (see Bagshawe et al,

---

[2] Radiochemical Centre, Amersham.

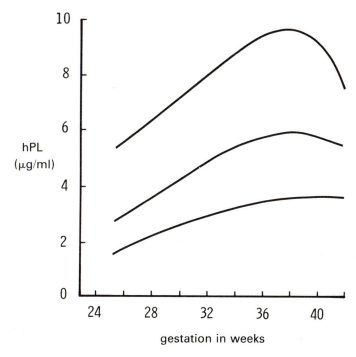

Fig. 6.1. A normal range of hPL. Note that the distribution around the mean is skewed (see Chap. 3).

1979). Neither application fits into the usual category of a 'placental function test', and they will not be considered further here.

Quantitative measurement of hCG has also been widely advocated as a test for the wellbeing of an early pregnancy. Two clinical areas have been defined: prognosis of threatened abortion and differential diagnosis of ectopic pregnancy.

Threatened abortion. In cases of vaginal bleeding of uncertain significance measurement of hCG levels may be of considerable prognostic value. In one study on a total of 148 patients, abnormally low serum hCG concentrations were found in 86% of the 89 women who subsequently aborted, but in none of the 59 patients with a satisfactory outcome (Dhont et al. 1975). In a similar study of 188 patients, normal levels of hCG were associated with a satisfactory outcome in 92% of cases (Jouppila et al. 1979). One problem in interpreting the literature on this topic is to assess the number of cases of 'unsatisfactory' outcome which were clinically obvious incomplete abortions at the time of first presentation.

A major problem in the practical use of hCG levels in early pregnancy is to establish the exact stage of gestation—obviously essential in deciding whether or not a result is normal. The levels change extremely rapidly from one week to the next; the doubling time of hCG in the first few weeks of pregnancy is

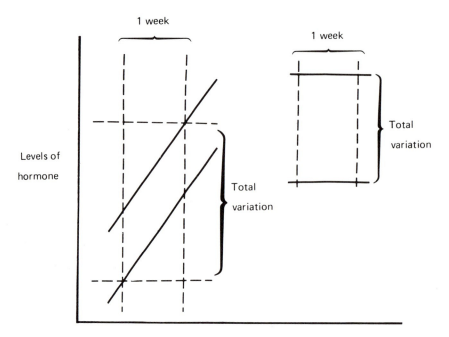

Fig. 6.2. The importance of errors in gestational dating in the interpretation of biochemical results. For a parameter which is rising rapidly (e.g. hCG in early pregnancy, oestrogens in late pregnancy) a 1-week gestational error (which is effectively the minimum in clinical practice) produces a large increase in the total variation (*left*). This effect is non-existent when the levels of the product are stable (*right*).

2–3 days. Thus a small clinical error in dating (e.g. 1 week) would make a critical difference to interpretation (Fig. 6.2) and may be one reason why the test is less than perfect. Equally, this also suggests that serial estimations may be of great value: if levels do not increase or actually fall over a period of 1 week, during which they would normally increase three-fold or more, then the pregnancy is likely to be abnormal.

Ectopic pregnancy. Using the sensitive RIA or the radioreceptor assay hCG levels are frequently positive in ectopic pregnancy (Seppälä et al. 1980). Seppälä et al. have shown that a rapid RIA is of value in the differential diagnosis of lower abdominal pain in women of reproductive age. In 100 such patients 24 gave a positive test and 22 of these had evidence of pregnancy, including 10 ectopics; of the 76 negative results only 3 had evidence of pregnancy.

hCG in late pregnancy

Because the levels fall after 12 weeks' gestation, hCG estimation has been little used for the monitoring of fetal wellbeing in late pregnancy. The rather

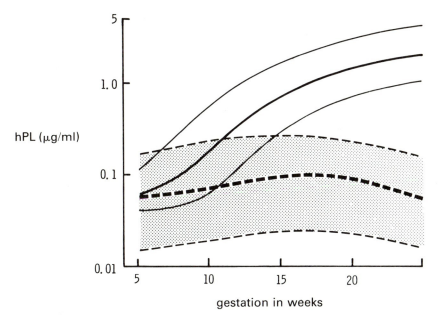

Fig. 6.3. Blood hPL levels in 141 subjects who aborted on first admission (*interrupted lines and hatched area*). The normal mean and range (± 2 SD) is shown by the *solid lines*.

sparse literature has been well summarised by Van Leusden (1976) and the general conclusion is that hCG assays in late pregnancy are not helpful in the management of late pregnancy complications.

hPL in early pregnancy

Though hPL measurements have been made in cases of trophoblastic tumour and, together with hCG, can provide a useful indication of the degree of malignancy, they are little used in routine clinical practice.

However, many authors have described the use of hPL in threatened abortion. The outcome for the fetus is uncertain in many cases of vaginal bleeding in early gestation and such patients may require several days of hospital admission before the final diagnosis is apparent. There is general agreement that low maternal hPL levels after the 8–10th week indicate that the outcome is likely to be unsatisfactory, and thus provide a valuable guide to prognosis in this condition (e.g. Niven et al. 1972) (Fig. 6.3). This applies whether or not a sonogram is also abnormal (Vorster et al. 1977). Low levels, and particularly serial low levels after the 10th week, would be an indication for evacuation of the uterus without further delay.

This information is very similar to that which can be obtained from hCG or SP1, though there is some evidence that both of these may be slightly more efficient than hPL before the 10th week of gestation.

hPL in late pregnancy

There is an extensive literature on maternal hPL levels in many of the complications of late pregnancy (see Letchworth 1976). These will be considered in turn.

Intrauterine growth retardation. Many workers have shown that hPL levels are correlated with the weight of the fetus (e.g. Letchworth et al. 1971). This relationship is secondary to that between the weight of the placenta and fetus, but there is general agreement that hPL levels are an efficient guide to fetal growth and prediction of delivery weight in an individual patient. The sensitivity of the test is around 40% (Morrison et al. 1980) and there are suggestions that it is still more efficient when the growth retardation is associated with maternal hypertension. Interestingly, it has also been shown that hPL levels are reduced in cases which can be described as growth retarded despite an apparently normal delivery weight (with reduced crown-heel length, reduced head circumference, etc.) (Daikoku et al. 1979). As might be expected twins have higher hPL values (Garoff and Seppälä 1973) but because the normal values for twins week by week are not known, it is impossible to say whether growth-retarded twins have lower hPL values than their normally grown counterparts.

Pre-eclampsia and hypertension. Spellacy et al. (1971) described a 'fetal danger zone' for subjects with hypertension: values of less than 4 µg/ml after the 30th week indicated a fetal mortality of 24%. The levels are generally lower in multigravidae than in primigravidae and it has been suggested that the greatest risk and lowest levels are associated with chronic vascular disease. Other workers have shown a similar clear association between low hPL levels and fetal outcome (Keller et al. 1971). Kelly et al. (1975) showed a 75% fetal risk (growth retardation or perinatal asphyxia) for subjects developing hypertension after the 28th week and having hPL concentrations less than two standard deviations below the normal mean.

The somewhat confusing literature on hPL levels in pre-eclampsia can be attributed to two factors. First, that the condition itself is very heterogeneous and is often not clearly defined. Second, that it is all too common for authors not to distinguish between pre-eclampsia per se, and the fetal risk arising from the pre-eclampsia. Thus, it is our impression that maternal hPL levels relate closely to the growth and development of the fetus and that this relationship is independent of other complications. In other words, hPL levels in the mother of a growth-retarded 2.3-kg fetus would be essentially the same whether or not there was a specific cause such as pre-eclampsia.

Diabetic mothers. Since diabetes mellitus is associated with a large placenta it would be expected that hPL would be generally elevated in this condition. This has been confirmed by numerous workers (e.g. Ursell et al. 1973) (Fig. 6.4). The levels are reduced in cases in which fetal outcome is unsatisfactory (Fig 6.5). Thus hPL levels in diabetic pregnancies must be interpreted in relation to the elevated range for 'normal diabetics'. While under most circumstances a level of 4 μg/ml is a useful dividing line for the diagnosis of abnormality, in patients with diabetes the critical level becomes 5 μg/ml.

Some conflicting results on the clinical value of hPL levels can be attributed to a number of factors, including the definition of the severity of the condition, the failure to appreciate that abnormality should be judged in relation to the general elevation of levels in this condition, and the fact that perinatal death may occur due to metabolic dysfunction in the absence of notable placental deficiency.

Rhesus isoimmunisation. Most workers have agreed that hPL levels are generally elevated in this condition, but few have found this to be of clinical value. However, one group has shown that the levels are most elevated when the child is severely affected (Ward et al. 1974) (Fig. 6.6). Before the 26th week, a value which is greater than two standard deviations above the normal

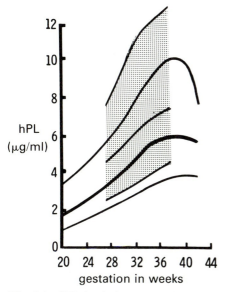

Fig. 6.4. hPL levels in pregnancies complicated by diabetes mellitus in which there was no evidence of placental dysfunction. The normal range is shown by *solid lines*.

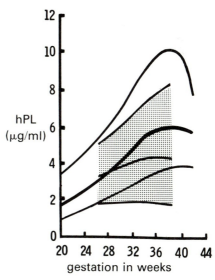

Fig. 6.5. hPL levels in pregnancies complicated by diabetes mellitus in which there was evidence of placental dysfunction. The normal range is shown by *solid lines*.

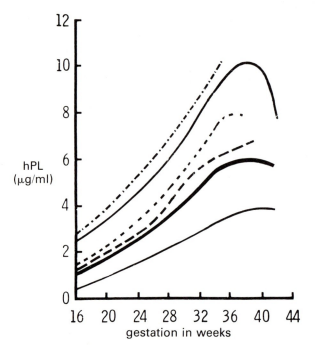

Fig. 6.6. Mean hPL levels in pregnancies complicated by Rhesus-isoimmunisation: ·—·— severely affected cases; ------ moderately affected cases; ——— mild cases.

mean indicates a 90% likelihood that the case will be severe. Similar elevations are seen in amniotic fluid hPL. Thus, the test may provide an additional diagnostic aid at a stage when other parameters, such as liquor bilirubin, may be equivocal.

Fetal death. In many cases hPL levels fall before fetal death occurs. This is in agreement with the fact that in many stillbirths the primary cause is placental insufficiency; only rarely does the primary cause lie within the fetus itself. Predictive value appears to be excellent. In one series of hypertensive patients low hPL levels correctly predicted 13 or 14 stillbirths (Spellacy et al. 1971).

Fetal distress and neonatal asphyxia. The literature on this subject is confused. Some authors have found an apparently good relationship between serial hPL levels and fetal complications occurring either during labour or at the time of delivery (e.g. Letchworth and Chard 1972). Thus a patient who is otherwise normal and who has three or more levels below 4 μg/ml in the last 6 weeks of pregnancy has a 71% risk of fetal complications. However, other authors have not found a relationship between hPL and acute events during labour (Seppälä and Ruoslahti 1970). Much of the confusion probably arises from the selection of clinical materials. Acute problems during labour may occur in a pregnancy which was perfectly normal up to that time. The inclusion of many such cases would detract from the apparent value of a placental function test which can only identify the more chronic problems. Thus hPL should only be able to predict those cases of acute fetal distress which are based on long-term placental insufficiency, and it is of interest to note that the most favourable figures in respect of fetal distress or evidence of neonatal asphyxia (sensitivity 87%; Morrison et al. 1980) were obtained from a group of growth-retarded infants.

Prolonged pregnancy. Maternal blood and amniotic fluid levels of hPL decrease in prolonged pregnancy (43 weeks and more) (Lolis et al. 1977). Whether low values serve to define a special 'at risk' group or merely indicate a general decline of placental function in postmaturity, is uncertain.

Other conditions. Maternal blood hPL levels are generally lower in smokers than in non-smokers; the effect seems to be directly related to the fetal growth retardation which is characteristic of these cases (Lee et al. 1980).

Conclusions—hPL levels in the management of late pregnancy

As a classic placental function test maternal hPL levels are widely used in routine obstetric care, especially in Europe. The only immediately obvious competition to hPL is the oestrogen assay, and there is little to suggest that one is better than the other. In any case comparisons are unreal as they represent very different physiological entities. Other placental proteins such as SP1 may be more fairly compared, but little is known about the changes of SP1 in obstetric disease compared to the voluminous literature on hPL.

Because maternal hPL is a convenient and well-established test it has been the subject of several excellent studies which set out to define its overall place in obstetric measurement. For example, Grudzinskas et al. (1981) used a 'relative risk factor' to demonstrate that low hPL levels, observed as part of a routine screening programme on an entire obstetric population, were as effective a predictor of poor fetal outcome as the occurrence of severe pre-eclampsia, low maternal weight at 32 weeks, and heavy smoking by the mother. All were superior to many other factors which are widely considered to be of great value in antenatal diagnosis. In an earlier study from Spellacy et al. (1975), hPL estimations were carried out on a large number of at-risk subjects; the patients were divided into two randomised groups, in one of which the results were reported to the clinicians and in the other they were not. In the first group the perinatal death rate was 3.4%, in the second 15%, an indication of the real practical value of these determinations. Given the fact that a substantial proportion of perinatal mortality and morbidity cannot be identified by existing clinical procedures, and that specificity (prediction of normal outcome) of other procedures is no better than that of hPL, a good argument can be made for the routine application of hPL measurement or a comparable determination in all pregnancies.

References

Aschheim S, Zondek B (1927) Hypophysen vorderlappenhormon und ovarialhormon im Harn von Schwangeren. Link Wschr 6: 1322
Bagshawe KD, Searle F, Wass M (1979) Human chorionic gonadotrophin. In: Gray CH, James VHT (eds) Hormones in blood. Academic Press, London, pp 364–411
Chard T (1979) Human placental lactogen. In: Gray CH, James VHT (eds) Hormones in blood. Academic Press, London, pp 333–363
Chard T (1981) Synthesis of placental lactogen by human placentae. In: Fotherby K, Pal SB (eds) Hormones in normal and abnormal human tissues, vol I. Walter de Gruyter, Berlin, pp 409–428
Daikoku NH, Tyson JE, Graf C, Scott R, Smith B, Johnston JWC, King TM (1979) The relative significance of human placental lactogen in the diagnosis of retarded fetal growth. J Obst Gynecol 135: 516
Dhont M, Thiery M, Vandekerckhove D, van Cauwenberghe A (1975) Klinische waarde van de radioimmunoassay van placentaire eiwithormonen in der verloskunde. Tijdschr voor Geneesk 22: 1097
Ehrhardt K (1936) Über das Laktations Hormon des Hypophysen-Vorderlappens. Münch Med Wschr 83: 1163
Garoff L, Seppälä M (1973) Alphafetoprotein and human placental lactogen levels in maternal serum in multiple pregnancies. Br J Obstet Gynaecol 86: 695–700
Gaspard U (1980) Les hormones protéiques placentaires. Masson, Paris
Grudzinskas JG, Gordon YB, Wadsworth J, Menabawey M, Chard T (1981) Is placental function testing worthwhile? An update on placental lactogen. Aust NZ J Obstet Gynaecol 21: 103
Ito Y, Higashi K (1961) Studies on the prolactin-like substance in human placenta. Endocrinol Jpn 8: 279
Josimovich JB, MacLaren JA, (1962) Presence in the human placenta and term serum of a highly lactogenic substance immunologically related to pituitary growth hormone. Endocrinology 71: 209
Jouppila P, Tapanainen J, Huhtanieni I (1979) Plasma hCG levels in patients with bleeding in the first and second trimesters of pregnancy. Br J Obstet Gynaecol 86; 343
Keller PJ, Bader P, Schmid J, Baertschi U, Gerber C, Soltermann R, Kopper E (1971) Biochemical detection of fetoplacental distress in risk pregnancies. Lancet ii: 729
Kelly AM, England P, Lorimer JD, Fergusson JC, Govan ADT (1975) An evaluation of human placental lactogen levels in hypertension of pregnancy. Br J Obstet Gynaecol 82: 272
Lee JN, Grudzinskas JG, Chard T (1980) Circulating placental lactogen (hPL) levels in relation to smoking during pregnancy. J Obstet Gynaecol 1: 87
Letchworth AT (1976) Human placental lactogen assay as a guide to fetal well-being. In: Klopper A (ed) Plasma hormone assays in evaluation of fetal wellbeing. Churchill Livingstone, Edinburgh, pp 147–173
Letchworth AT, Chard T (1972) Placental lactogen levels as a screening test for fetal distress and neonatal asphyxia. Lancet i: 704
Letchworth AT, Boardman RJ, Bristow C, Landon J, Chard T (1971) A rapid semi-automated method for the measurement of human chorionic somatomammotrophin. The normal range in the third trimester and its relation to fetal weight. J Obstet Gynaecol Br Commonwealth 78: 542
Lolis, D, Konstantinidis K, Paperangelou G, Kaskarelis D (1977) Comparative study of amniotic fluid and maternal blood serum hormone placental lactogen in normal and prolonged pregnancies. J Obstet Gynecol 128: 724

References

Morrison I, Green P, Oomen B (1980) The role of human placental lactogen assays in antepartum fetal assessment. Am J Obstet Gynecol 136: 1055

Nielsen PV, Pedersen H, Kampmann E-M (1979) Absence of human placental lactogen in an otherwise uneventful pregnancy. Am J Obstet Gynecol 135: 322

Niven PAR, Landon J, Chard T (1972) Placental lactogen levels as a guide to outcome of threatened abortion. Br Med J ii: 799

Pavlou C, Chard T, Letchworth AT (1972) Circulating levels of human chorionic somatomammotrophin in late pregnancy: disappearance from the circulation after delivery, variation during labour, and circadian variation. J Obstet Gynaecol Br Commonwealth 79: 629

Samaan N, Gallagher H, McRoberts W, Farris A (1971) Serial estimations of human placental lactogen (hPL), estriol and pregnanediol in pregnancy correlated with whole organ section of placenta. Am J Obstet Gynecol 109: 53–73

Saxena BB, Hasan SH, Haour F, Gollwitzer MS (1974) Radioreceptor assay of human chorionic gonadotrophin: Early detection of pregnancy. Science 184: 793

Seppälä M, Ruoslahti E (1970) Serum concentrations of human placental lactogenic hormone (hPL) in pregnancy complications. Acta Obstet Gynecol Scand 49: 143–147

Seppälä M, Tontti K, Ranta T, Stenman UH, Chard T (1980) Use of a rapid hCG-beta-subunit radioimmunoassay in acute gynaecological emergencies. Lancet i: 165

Spellacy WN, Teoh ES, Buhi WC, Birk SA, McCreary SA (1971) Value of human chorionic somatomammotropin in managing high-risk pregnancies. Am J Obstet Gynecol 109: 588

Spellacy WN, Buhi WC, Birk SA (1975) The effectiveness of human placental lactogen as an adjunct in decreasing perinatal deaths. Am J Obstet Gynecol 121: 835

Ursell W, Brudenell M, Chard T (1973) Placental lactogen levels in diabetic pregnancy. Br Med J ii: 80

Van Leusden HA (1976) Chorionic gonadotrophin in pathological pregnancy. In: Klopper A (ed) hormone assays in evaluation of fetal wellbeing. Churchill Livingstone, Edinburgh, pp 48–71

Vorster CZ, Pannall PR, Slabber CF (1977) The prognostic value of serum human placental lactogen determinations in early pregnancy. Am J Obstet Gynecol 128: 879

Ward RHT, Letchworth AT, Niven PAR, Chard T (1974) Placental lactogen levels in Rhesus iso-immunisation. Br Med J i: 347

Chapter 7
Other Placental Proteins

In the last decade several new proteins of placental origin have been discovered in the maternal circulation. Their concentration increases during gestation *pari passu* with placental growth in much the same way as hPL. As their physiological role is unknown they cannot be classed as hormones. This is largely a matter of how a hormone is defined; in the broadest sense some of them may prove to be hormones. From the point of view of placental function tests, this is irrelevant: their rising concentration may reflect placental growth and function and that is our sole concern.

Discovery of new placental proteins

The first of the new placental proteins was discovered independently in Moscow, in Marburg and in Miami. All the discoveries resulted from the application of a routine immunological technique: injection of whole pregnancy serum into rabbits, resulting in an array of antibodies to the serum proteins of a pregnant woman. If such an antiserum is absorbed with non-pregnancy serum the remaining antibodies are to proteins peculiar to pregnancy or much increased during pregnancy. The latter include such proteins as sex-hormone-binding globulin, pregnancy zone protein (like sex-hormone-binding globulin a protein whose production by the maternal liver is stimulated by rising oestrogen concentrations) and alphafetoprotein. This technique led to the discovery of a number of new proteins peculiar to pregnancy and presumed to originate from the placenta. The number of such proteins already runs into double figures and more are being reported every month. This account will be limited to the four about which placental function studies have been published. Most investigators named the proteins which they discovered, generally in terms of the physicochemical characteristics which had enabled their isolation, and only later found that their protein had been given a name by a previous investigator. This confusion has been somewhat cleared up by an agreed nomenclature (Halbert 1979). Table 7.1 lists the proteins, with their synonyms, which will be considered in this chapter.

Table 7.1. Pregnancy-'specific' plasma proteins

Preferred designation	Reference	Alternative name
1. SP1 (Schwangerschaftspezifisches protein 1)	Bohn 1971	Trophoblastic-specific β_1-globulin PAPP-C (pregnancy-associated plasma protein C) PSβG (pregnancy-specific β_1-glycoprotein)
2. PAPP-A (pregnancy-associated plasma protein A)	Lin et al. 1974	
3. PAPP-B (pregnancy-associated plasma protein B)	Lin et al. 1974	
4. PP5 (placental protein 5)	Bohn and Winckler 1977	

Schwangerschaftsprotein 1 (SP1)

Although this protein was first isolated by Tatarinov and Masyukevich (1970) and subsequently by Bohn (1971) and by Gall and Halbert (1972) the first clear description of its physicochemical characteristics came from Bohn's laboratory in Marburg. He determined that SP1 had a molecular weight of 90,000 daltons and the electrophoretic mobility of a β_1-globulin. A large part (30%) of the molecule consisted of carbohydrate containing sialic acid. The amino acid sequence has not been studied and it is therefore impossible to determine whether it resembles any other known protein. It does not appear to have common antigenic determinants with other known placental proteins and its biological activity, if any, is unknown.

There is no doubt about the identity of the protein originally described by Bohn (1971) but it is now apparent that pregnancy serum contains a second protein which cross-reacts with antisera to SP1 (Teisner et al. 1978, 1979a). This second protein is larger (400,000 daltons) and has α_2-electrophoretic mobility. The nomenclature has therefore to be revised: the original molecule being designated SP1ß and Teisner's new molecule SP1α, the term SP1 being reserved for a mixture of the two. It has been shown that SP1α is formed by the combination of SP1ß with a second protein (Bohn 1979; Ahmed and Klopper 1980). The protein with which SP1ß combines to form SP1α is not of placental origin but occurs in the blood of non-pregnant individuals (Ahmed et al. 1980).

Synthesis

SP1ß has been located in the syncytiotrophoblast by immunofluorescent staining (Lin and Halbert 1976) and placental tissue incorporates radioactivity from labelled amino acids into protein with SP1 immunological determinants (Horne et al. 1976). SP1α can also be extracted from the placenta but is much more tightly bound and requires Triton X100 to solubilise it in placental homogenates (Ahmed et al. 1980). A reasonable hypothesis is that in binding with a serum protein to form SP1α, the SP1ß becomes firmly attached to insoluble trophoblastic constituents, some of which escape into the maternal circulation and exist as an equilibrium mixture with SP1α. It follows that all pregnancy sera must contain some SP1α. It is not commonly detected because immunoprecipitates of SP1α require treatment with polyethylene glycol to be visualised.

Measurement

In late pregnancy SP1 is present in high concentration in maternal plasma, about 20 times that of hPL (Klopper et al. 1977). It is therefore easy to measure by simple, insensitive immunoprecipitation methods such as the radial immunodiffusion (Mancini) technique. The first placental function studies were done by this method. The second wave of clinical studies used the more sensitive rocket immunoelectrophoresis of the Laurell type (Bruce and Klopper 1978). Even this could not measure SP1 earlier than 15–20 weeks' gestation, so RIA methods were evolved (Grudzinskas et al. 1977).

It is not possible to make firm recommendations about methods of assay in view of the confusion created by the discovery of two separate proteins reacting with SP1 antisera. RIA measures SP1β almost exclusively in physiologial mixtures of SP1α and SP1β because of the use of relatively pure SP1β tracers (Teisner et al. 1979b). This begs the question of what constitutes a physiological mixture and will depend on the particular antiserum. Techniques are evolving fast and once the combining protein is isolated, it should be possible to make an antiserum which is specific for SP1α or, alternatively, to separate SP1α and SP1β before estimation with an SP1 antiserum.

Variability

SP1 has a long half-life in the maternal circulation; 22 h as compared with 15 min for hPL (Klopper et al. 1978). The average coefficient of variation from day to day is 5%, much of which can be accounted for in terms of methodological variability (Masson et al. 1977). This steadiness has much to recommend it in terms of placental function studies. Although the response to deterioration in placental function may be slow, so also is the development of placental malfunction which may set the fetus at risk. As with other placental products the subject-to-subject variation is large, so that there is likely to be considerable overlap between low normal values and the highest pathological results. In one study the subject-to-subject coefficient of variation was 30% at 38 weeks' gestation. In the same subjects at this time the variability in hPL concentration was 36% (Klopper et al. 1979).

Normal range

The normal range for SP1 in late pregnancy as recorded by various investigators is shown in Table 7.2. None can be regarded as definitive until SP1α and SP1β are measured separately against authentic standards by specific methods. In the meantime it is essential that each laboratory should establish its own standard.

Table 7.2 Circulating levels of SP1 in late pregnancy. Note the wide range of levels due to use of different assay methods and standards. RID, radial immunodiffusion; RIA, radioimmunoassay; EID, electroimmunidiffusion ('rocket' immunoelectrophoresis)

Author	No. of subjects	Mean (mg/litre)	S.D.	Coefficient of variation	Method of assay
Tatra et al.	22	139	42.5	30.6	RID
Towler et al. 1976	16	199	53.9	27.1	RID
Gordon et al. 1977	59	250	—	9[a]	RIA
Klopper et al. 1978	53	159	48.0	30.2	RID
Lin et al. 1974	41	2200 U/litre	—	—	RID
Sorensen 1978	20	199	—	—	EID

[a]This figure was calculated after logarithmic transformation of results. As a skewed distribution appears to be universal for all placental proteins including SP1, analysis as arithmetic mean and standard deviations is probably not valid. A non-parametric analysis (median and centiles) is the best approach.

Clinical applications of SP1 measurement

Early pregnancy

SP1 appears in the maternal circulation very early in pregnancy, at least as soon as hCG (Grudzinskas et al. 1977). The main application of SP1 assay may be as a pregnancy test since low levels of hCG are easily confused with LH. The use of SP1 assays as a monitor for trophoblastic tumours has not been examined in detail but the initial publications suggest that it has promise.

Measurement of SP1 has been put forward as a test for the prognosis of threatened abortion. The good results achieved in some investigations may be deceptive. Many of the assays were done on patients in whom the abortion process was already well advanced and where the clinician would have been in little doubt as to the correct management. The same does not apply to the largest series of 245 cases, reported by Jouppila et al. (1980). They found the sensitivity of the test to be 65% and the predictive value 96% (Fig. 7.1).

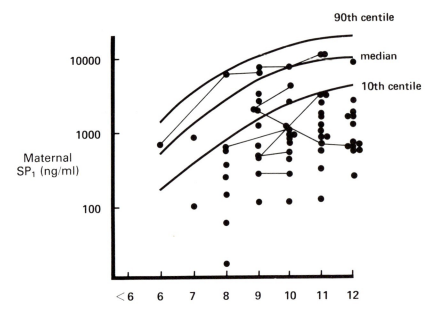

Fig. 7.1. Maternal serum SP1 levels in patients with clinical signs of threatened abortion in whom the pregnancy subsequently aborted.

These figures are at least as good as those reported for other parameters, including biochemical markers such as hCG and hPL, and ultrasound examination.

Intrauterine growth retardation

Many investigators have found that low birthweight for gestation is frequently accompanied by low levels of SP1 (Lin et al. 1976; Gordon et al. 1977; Towler et al. 1977; Chapman and Jones 1978; Sorensen 1978). In two such studies low levels were found in 70% and 60% of cases in which the birthweight of the child was less than the 10th centile of the normal population (Chapman and Jones 1978; Gordon et al. 1977). The test may also have predictive value in mid-trimester (Salem et al. 1981b). Presumably the low SP1 values result from retarded placental growth and are only indirectly related to fetal growth retardation. Retarded fetal growth is not a homogeneous entity but the results do not seem to vary with the cause of the growth retardation (Fig. 7.2). None of the investigators have analysed their findings in terms of the risk factors suggested in Chap. 3. Until this is done it is very difficult to assess the true value of SP1 assays in retarded fetal growth, particularly in comparison with other parameters such as oestriol or hPL measurements.

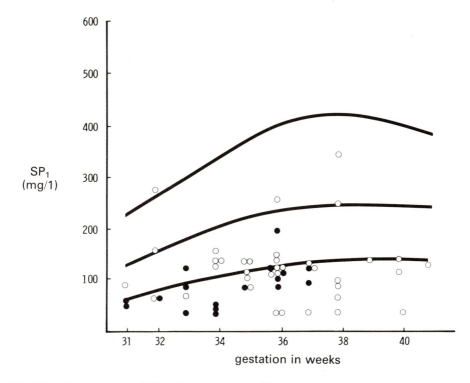

Fig. 7.2. Maternal serum SP1 levels in patients with (●) and without (○) hypertension in whom there was growth retardation of the fetus. The *solid lines* show the median and 10th and 90th centiles of the normal range.

Pre-eclampsia and hypertension

The levels of SP1 in hypertensive disorders of pregnancy seem to relate to the presence or absence of fetal complications rather than to the condition itself (Chapman and Jones 1978). (Fig. 7.2).

Diabetic mothers

The only substantial study on this subject reported normal levels in a group of 20 diabetic subjects (Grudzinskas et al. 1979). These findings are somewhat unexpected in the light of previous observations to the effect that levels of placental proteins are elevated in diabetes mellitus. It may be, however, that the diabetes in the study group was so well controlled that they effectively had normal pregnancies. It is now a major problem of research into diabetic pregnancy; the uncontrolled diabetic is a thing of the past.

Assessment of placental function

Except for its longer half-life and higher concentration SP1 closely resembles hPL, and it may be that assays of SP1 will be used for much the same purpose. In late pregnancy the simplicity of the assay is a great advantage. In early pregnancy SP1 assays are more informative than those for hPL. This may be due to nothing more than its higher concentration. The true clinical value of assays of SP1 may not be known until it is possible to assess SP1β and SP1α separately.

Placental protein 5 (PP5)

PP5 was first isolated from the placenta by Bohn in 1972. Subsequent publications from the same laboratory (Bohn and Winckler 1977) showed it to be a β_1-globulin with a molecular weight of 36,000 and a carbohydrate content of 12%. There is evidence to suggest that, like SP1, there may be more than one molecular species with PP5 antigenic determinants (Salem et al. 1980).

Physiology

PP5 has a short half-life, 5–38 min, of the same order as hPL (Obiekwe et al., in preparation). Its concentration in maternal blood is much lower than that of SP1 and it can only be measured by RIA (Obiekwe et al. 1979).

PP5 exists in blood in both low and high molecular weight forms; the values in serum are significantly higher than in plasma (Salem et al. 1980). The explanation may be that it is associated with coagulation. Early studies showed that it could act as an enzyme inhibitor (Bohn and Winckler 1977). Recently it has been shown that PP5 can form complexes with heparin (Salem et al. 1981a), that it interacts with thrombin (Salem et al. 1981b) and that it shows a unique pattern of changes in obstetric pathology known to be associated with coagulation abnormalities (Salem et al. 1981c). Current speculation proposes that PP5 is closely related to antithrombin III and might, therefore, act as a natural anticoagulant at the placental site. There is, however, no evidence concerning the control and mechanism of PP5 production.

Clinical applications of PP5 measurement

PP5 assays have not been used in early pregnancy; the concentration is too low for routine measurements, even by RIA. In late pregnancy PP5 levels are related to fetal weight (Obiekwe et al. 1980). It is, however, not a useful test for fetal growth retardation as the sensitivity is only 17%—considerably less than that of either SP1 or hPL. A very interesting potential application is the observation that *elevated* levels may be associated with placental abruption and that the test may indeed have predictive value in this respect (Salem et al. 1981c) (Fig. 7.3), a possibility that fits with its putative role in placental coagulation. A further finding of interest is that PP5 levels measured at 16 weeks' gestation are predictive of premature labour—an objective which at present can be achieved by no other obstetric parameter (Salem et al. 1981b).

These hints of a physiological role in placental homeostasis put PP5 in a different category from hPL and SP1. Simply as an index of placental mass it is clearly not as useful as either of the other two proteins. If, however, it plays a vital role in placental processes not connected with fetal growth, quite different possibilities of clinical application arise. Certainly the measurement of PP5 deserves much closer study.

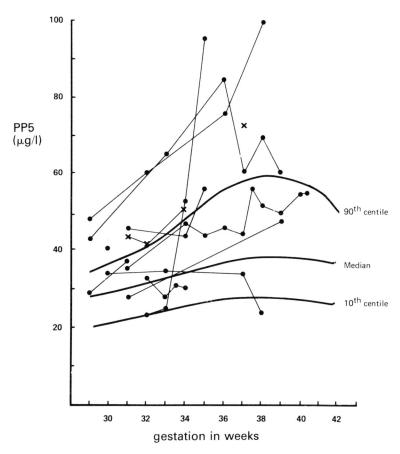

Fig. 7.3. Maternal serum PP5 levels in serial samples from patients with placental abruption (●———● singleton; x———x twins).

Pregnancy-associated plasma protein A (PAPP-A)

The Miami team isolated four proteins from the blood of pregnant women which could not be found in males or non-pregnant women (Lin et al. 1974). They named them pregnancy-associated plasma proteins A, B, C and D. It was later shown that PAPP-C was SP1 and PAPP-D was hPL. They measured normal levels of PAPP-A and PAPP-B and examined their relationship to various characteristics of pregnancy (Lin et al. 1976) and explored the clinical applications of their assay (Lin et al. 1977), but in spite of some very promising findings these assays were not taken up elsewhere until recently. Very little is known about PAPP-B and we do not propose to consider it further. The findings with regard to PAPP-A are intriguing and bear further examination.

Chemistry

PAPP-A is a glycoprotein containing sialic acid (Lin et al. 1974). It is a macroglobulin with α_2-electrophoretic mobility and has a molecular weight of 750,000–820,000. Bischof (1979) has suggested that it is a dimer with each monomer being composed of two polypeptide chains of 218,000 daltons. Thus in many ways it resembles α_2-macroglobulin, although there is no immunological cross-reaction between them. Although it is now possible to get clean preparations of PAPP-A by relatively simple immunoabsorption techniques, the initial purifications from pregnancy serum were laborious and involved ammonium sulphate precipitation, ion-exchange chromatography, affinity chromatography on Concanavalin-A and gel filtration. Even the immunological techniques yield barely enough pure protein for simple investigation of its biological properties.

Synthesis

Immunofluorescent studies located PAPP-A in the cytoplasm of the villous trophoblast (Lin and Halbert 1976) but later investigations have cast some doubt on this. Thus, there is stronger PAPP-A immunofluorescence in the perivillous fibrin (Page Faulk, personal communication), and Klopper et al. (1979) found lower concentrations of PAPP-A in the retroplacental blood than in the uterine vein or peripheral veins. It is possible that PAPP-A reaches the maternal circulation, not by secretion from the villous syncytiotrophoblast, but by dissolution of migrating trophoblast, or even that it is produced in the decidua and absorbed by the trophoblast. This raises the possibility that PAPP-A may be a maternal rather than a fetal protein. If true, the physiology of PAPP-A and the use of assays of PAPP-A as a test of placental function must be re-examined.

Measurement

In late pregnancy the concentration of PAPP-A is sufficiently high for the protein to be measured by immunoelectrophoresis (Bischof et al. 1979). RIAs capable of measuring PAPP-A in early pregnancy are only now coming into use and as yet little is known about early pregnancy values. No pure standard of PAPP-A is available and measurements are made in terms of arbitrary units as defined by the PAPP-A content of a sample of pooled late pregnancy serum held by the World Health Organisation in Lyons, France.

Metabolism

PAPP-A has a half-life of 18 h (Klopper et al. 1978). This is based on the rate of decline of PAPP-A in plasma after delivery of the placenta and assumes that all sources of input of PAPP-A are removed with the placenta. If PAPP-A enters the maternal circulation from a different point this figure would be seriously in error and PAPP-A may have a much shorter half-life.

Variability

The subject-to-subject spread of PAPP-A is of the order of 30% (Klopper et al. 1979). The distribution is skewed, being extended by a few extremely high values. The normal range, therefore, is best described in non-parametric terms, i.e. as a median and centiles. Like other placental proteins such as hPL and SP1, the day-to-day variability of PAPP-A is about 5%, and in this respect compares favourably with the steroids.

Normal range

After 12 weeks PAPP-A rises steadily. Other placental products such as hPL and SP1 tend to flatten out at 36–40 weeks as the increase in functional trophoblastic tissue slows and stops. Some uncertain evidence suggests that PAPP-A tends to continue rising right up to term—another indication that PAPP-A is not simply related to placental mass. If, indeed, PAPP-A continues to rise right up to term then clinical interpretation should be based on failure of the normal rise rather than comparison with the normal range for a given week.

The value of PAPP-A measurements in late pregnancy, as with other parameters, is related to the cause of the fetal hazard. There have been claims (Lin et al. 1976) that PAPP-A levels are related to placental and fetal size. However, others have not confirmed a relationship between PAPP-A concentration and fetal weight, and the measurements do not appear to be useful in the diagnosis or management of retarded fetal growth (Bischof et al. 1981).

One very interesting clinical application of PAPP-A assays is becoming apparent. Halbert and Lin (1979) found that the concentration was increased in pre-eclamptic toxaemia. This was confirmed by Hughes et al. (1980a), who also suggested that a rise in PAPP-A often precedes the overt signs of the disease. The use of PAPP-A assays as a screen for pre-eclampsia was confirmed by Toop and Klopper (1981). There is also some evidence to suggest that the assays could be useful in antepartum haemorrhage and premature labour (Hughes et al. 1980b), findings similar to those with PP5. PAPP-A assays are likely to be more useful as an antenatal screening measure than as a device for detecting rapidly deteriorating placental function.

We have already put forward the thesis that in many respects placental products derive their relationship to fetal wellbeing simply by reflecting placental blood flow. Viewed in this light PAPP-A measurements are not useful and cannot compete with established parameters such as hPL. Placental blood flow is reduced in pre-eclampsia: PAPP-A is not; on the contrary, it is raised before onset of the disease. It might well be related to the genesis of the condition which puts its measurement in quite a different category. The best evidence regarding the role of PAPP-A in pregnancy shows that it is an inhibitor of complement fixation. Its connection with pre-eclamptic toxaemia may therefore be immunological.

References

Ahmed AG, Klopper A (1980) Separation of two pregnancy-associated proteins with SP1 determinants and the conversion of SP1α to SP1β. Arch Gynecol 280: 95–108

Ahmed AG, Toop K, Klopper A (1980) The demonstration of two pregnancy-associated proteins with SP1 determinants in placental extracts. Placenta 2: 45–52

Bischof P (1979) Purification and characterisation of pregnancy-associated plasma protein A (PAPP-A). Arch Gynecol 227: 315–321

Bischof P, Bruce D, Dunnigham P, Klopper A (1979) Measurement of pregnancy-associated plasma protein A (PAPP-A). Clin Chim Acta 95: 243–247

Bischof P, Hughes G, Klopper A (1981) Relationship of obstetric parameters to the concentration of pregnancy-associated plasma protein A (PAPP-A). Am J Obstet Gynecol 138: 494–499

Bohn H (1971) Nachweis und Charakterisierung von Schwangerschaftsproteinen in der menschlichen Plazenta sowie ihre quantitative immunologische Bestimmung im Serum schwangerer Frauen. Arch Gynaekol 210: 440–457

Bohn H (1979) Placental and pregnancy proteins. In: Lehmann F (ed) Carcino-embryonic proteins. Elsevier/North-Holland, Amsterdam, pp 294–295

Bohn H, Winckler W (1977) Isolierung und Charakteriserung eines neuen Gewebsproteins, PP5. Arch Gynakol 223: 179–186

Bruce D, Klopper A (1978) The measurement of pregnancy-specific β_1 glycoprotein by electroimmunodiffusion. Clin Chim Acta 84: 107–113

Chapman MG, Jones WR (1978) Pregnancy-specific β_1 glycoprotein (SP-1) in normal and abnormal pregnancy. Aust NZ J Obstet Gynaecol 18: 172

Gall SA, Halbert SP (1972) Antigenic constituents in pregnancy plasma which are undetectable in normal non-pregnant female or male plasma. Int Arch Allergy Appl Immunol 42: 503-515

Gordon YB, Grudzinskas JG, Jeffrey D, Chard T, Letchworth AT (1977) Concentrations of pregnancy-specific β_1 glycoprotein in normal pregnancy and in intrauterine growth retardation. Lancet i: 331-333

References

Grudzinskas JG, Gordon YB, Jeffrey D, Chard T (1977) Specific and sensitive determination of pregnancy specific β_1 glycoprotein (SP1) by radioimmunoassay: A new pregnancy test. Lancet i: 333–335

Grudzinskas JG, Gordon YB, Davies JH, Brudenell M, Chard T (1979) Circulating levels of pregnancy specific glycoprotein in pregnancies complicated by diabetes mellitus. Br J Obstet Gynaecol 86: 978

Halbert SP (1979) Nomenclature of pregnancy-'specific' plasma proteins. In: Klopper A, Chard T (eds) Placental proteins. Springer, Berlin, Heidelberg, New York, p 7

Halbert SP, Lin TM (1979) Pregnancy-associated plasma proteins: PAPP-A and PAPP-B. In: Klopper A, Chard T (eds) Placental proteins, Springer, Berlin, Heidelberg, New York, pp 89–104

Horne CW, Towler CM, Pugh-Humphreys RC, Thomson AW, Bohn H (1976). Pregnancy-specific β_1 glycoprotein—a product of the syncytiotrophoblast. Experientia 32: 1197–1199

Hughes G, Bischof P, Wilson G, Klopper A (1980a) Tests of fetal wellbeing in the third trimester of pregnancy. Br J Obstet Gynaecol 87: 650-656

Hughes G, Bischof P, Wilson G, Klopper A (1980b) Assay of a placental protein to determine fetal risk. Br Med J i: 671–673

Jouppila P, Seppälä M, Chard T (1980) Pregnancy-specific β_1 glycoprotein in complications of early pregnancy. Lancet i: 667

Klopper A, Masson G, Wilson G (1977) Plasma oestriol and placental proteins: A cross-sectional study at 38 weeks gestation. Br J Obstet Gynaecol 84: 648–655

Klopper A, Buchan P, Wilson G (1978) The puerperal decline of oestriol and pregnancy associated proteins. Br J Obstet Gynaecol 85: 738–747

Klopper A, Smith R, Davidson I (1979) The measurement of trophoblastic proteins as a test of placental function. In: Klopper A, Chard T (eds) Placental proteins. Springer, Berlin, Heidelberg, New York, pp 23–41

Lin TM, Halbert SP (1976) Placental localisation of human pregnancy-associated plasma proteins. Science 19: 1249–1252

Lin TM, Halbert SP, Keifer D, Spellacy W, Gall S (1974) Characterisation of four pregnancy-associated plasma proteins. Am J Obstet Gynecol 118: 223–226

Lin TM, Halbert SP, Spellacy W (1976) Relation of obstetric parameters to the concentrations of four pregnancy-associated plasma proteins at term in normal gestation. Am J Obstet Gynecol 125: 17–24

Lin TM, Halbert SP, Spellacy W, Berne BG (1977) Plasma concentrations of four pregnancy proteins in complications of pregnancy. Am J Obstet Gynecol 128: 808–810

Masson G, Klopper A, Wilson G (1977) Plasma oestrogens and pregnancy associated plasma proteins: A study of their variability in late pregnancy. Obstet Gynecol 50: 435–458

Obiekwe BC, Pendlebury DJ, Gordon YB, Grudzinskas JG, Chard T, Bohn H (1979) The radioimmunoassay of placental protein 5 and circulating levels in maternal blood in the third trimester of normal pregnancy. Clin Chim Acta 95: 509

Obiekwe BC, Grudzinskas JG, Chard T (1980) Circulating levels of placental protein 5 in the mother: relation to birthweight. Br J Obstet Gynaecol 87: 302–304

Salem HT, Obiekwe BC, Al-Ani ATM, Seppälä M, Chard T (1980) Molecular heterogeneity of placental protein 5 (PP5) in late pregnancy serum and plasma: evidence for a heparin-PP5 polymer. Clin Chim Acta 107: 211

Salem HT, Seppälä M, Chard T (1981a) The effect of thrombin on serum placental protein 5 (PP5): Is PP5 the naturally occurring antithrombin III of the human placenta? Placenta 2: 205

Salem HT, Lee JN, Seppälä M, Vaara L, Aula P, Al-Ani ATM, Chard T (1981b) Measurement of placental protein 5, placental lactogen and pregnancy specific β_1 glycoprotein in mid-trimester as a predictor of outcome of pregnancy. Br J Obstet Gynaecol 88: 371

Salem HT, Westergaard JG, Hindersson P, Seppälä M, Chard T (1981c) Placental protein 5 (PP5) in placental abruption. Br J Obstet Gynaecol 80: 500

Sorensen S (1979) An electroimmuno-assay of the pregnancy-specific β_1 glycoprotein (SP1) in normal and pathological pregnancies, and its clinical value compared to human chorionic somato-mammotropin (HCS). Acta Obstet Gynecol Scand 57: 201

Tatarinov YS, Masyukevich VN (1970) Immunological identification of a new beta 1-globulin in the blood serum of pregnant women. Biull Eksp Biol Med 69: 66–68

Tatra G, Breitenecker G, Gruber W (1974) Serum concentration of pregnancy-specific β_1

glycoprotein in normal and pathologic pregnancies. Arch Gynaekol 217: 383–390

Teisner B, Westergaard JG, Folkersen J, Husby S, Svehag L (1978). Two pregnancy-associated serum proteins with pregnancy-specific glycoprotein determinants. Am J Obstet Gynecol 131: 262–266

Teisner B, Folkersen J, Hindersson P, Jensenius J, Westergaard J (1979a) Quantification of the pregnancy-specific β_1 glycoprotein (SP1) by immunoprecipitation techniques. The influence of a cross-reacting high molecular weight α_2 protein. Scand J Immunol 9: 409–417

Teisner B, Grudzinskas JG, Hindersson O, Al-Ani ATM, Westergaard JG, Chard T (1979b) Molecular heterogeneity of pregnancy specific β_1 glycoprotein: The effect on measurement by radioimmunoassay and electroimmunoassay. J Immunol Methods 31: 141

Toop K, Klopper A (1981) Concentration of Pregnancy-associated Plasma Protein A (PAPP-A) in patients with pre-eclamptic toxaemia. In: Miller RK, Thiede H (eds) Placenta: Receptors, pathology and toxicology. Saunders, London, pp 167–171

Towler CM, Horne CH, Jandial V, Campbell DM, MacGillivray I (1976) Plasma levels of pregnancy-specific β_1 glycoprotein in normal pregnancy. Br J Obstet Gynaecol 83: 775–779

Towler CM, Horne CW, Jandial V, Campbell DM, MacGillivray I (1977) Plasma levels of pregnancy specific β_1 glycoprotein in complicated pregnancies. Br J Obstet Gynaecol 84: 258–263

Chapter 8
Conclusions: Choice and Use of Placental Function Tests

Having considered the nature of placental function tests and examined some test substances in detail it now remains to present some general conclusions. Of necessity these will report much of what has already been said, but the reader may find it useful to have the thread of the argument displayed without supporting data or any systematic marshalling of pros or cons. Three things are central to the use of biochemical tests of placental function: how the tests compare with other parameters of obstetric management; what value any test has in a specified abnormality of pregnancy; and which test is most helpful in obstetric management of particular abnormal states.

Placental function tests in antenatal care: are they worthwhile?

Antenatal care is a screening process. Trivial complaints apart, the null hypothesis of clinical obstetrics is that a pregnancy will be normal—an assumption correct in some 80%–90% of cases. All parameters are, in the first instance, designed to distinguish normality from abnormality. This contrasts with most other clinical testing, which is aimed at determining the degree of abnormality in situations where abnormality has already been defined—for example, cardiac function in a patient known to have mitral stenosis. Furthermore, the main point of placental function tests is to predict particular aspects of the outcome of a pregnancy rather than to diagnose a particular pathology. An abnormal placental function is not diagnostic of pre-eclampsia; but it might define the fetal risk in this condition.

The screening nature of most obstetric parameters must of itself blur attempts at comparison. But the situation is further confused by the fact that the relationship among different tests (tests, in this case, embracing the clinical, the electronic and the biochemical) is often unclear. It is quite possible, indeed common, for one parameter only to be abnormal: for a patient to have a history of a previous stillbirth, and an entirely normal pregnancy in every other respect; to have ultrasound evidence of growth retardation, in the absence of any other information to this effect. Thus, it is almost impossible to state with confidence that one test is 'better' than another when they are measuring different things, any one of which might be significant in an individual pregnancy.

Nevertheless, some perfectly reasonable attempts have been made to assess the overall place of placental function tests using the techniques described in Chap. 3. The most notable are those of Gorden et al. (1978) and Grudzinskas et al. (1981), and their findings are shown in detail in Table 8.1. This investigation is worthy of comment because it highlights several important points in the interpretation of any parameter used in obstetric care.

First, it illustrates the importance of studying a complete population to obtain meaningful comparisons. A test may appear to be good because it has a low incidence of false positives and false negatives. But if the condition the test is designed to reveal is rare then a very different picture emerges. Consider, for example, a condition with an incidence of 1%, and an associated test with a false negative rate of zero and a false positive rate of 10%. Superficially, the last two figures would appear excellent—yet a moment's reflection will reveal that in a complete population the test will give only one 'true' result for every ten 'positive' results. The type of analysis suggested by Gordon et al. (1978) is essential when using placental function tests as a means of screening the antenatal population. Using placental function tests in the individual woman is quite a different matter and the two should not be confused.

Second, the figures illustrate a pitfall in interpreting figures given for 'sensitivity'. For example, under the heading 'non-smokers' a figure of 55% is given, from which one might conclude that knowing a patient was a non-smoker is a useful test of fetal risk. The fallacy is that the positive test result (i.e. non-smoking) applies to most of the population—a factor which is immediately apparent when looking at the predictive value (8%) and relative risk (0.6). The reductio ad absurdum is that a test which was positive in the entire population (e.g. female sex of the mother) would have a sensitivity of 100%!

Third, the findings reveal an under-emphasised aspect of placental function tests: that they can upon occasion give a *positive* reassurance of fetal health, as witness the occurrence of high levels of hPL. Put another way, the facts accumulated in an antenatal clinic are usually divided into 'no news' (normal) and 'bad news' (abnormal). It is easy to forget that some observations are 'good news': that an hPL level above the 90th centile, in the absence of any other positive clinical findings, actually suggests that the pregnancy is better off than the remaining 90% of subjects.

Fourth, and finally, the figures give a pecking-order for the clinical significance of various observations made in antenatal care. If this population were completely representative of all other obstetric populations then certain conclusions could be reached. Detection of pre-eclampsia, fetal heart abnormalities, measurement of hPL and knowledge of maternal age, weight and smoking habits, are useful clinical tests. Other observations, such as social class, a history of stillbirth, or a history of threatened abortion, are of no statistically proven value. It is immediately obvious that the negative findings are a quirk of the small population (2069 subjects) examined. However, it is equally clear that a placental function test, in this case hPL, emerges with considerable credit when compared with other obstetric parameters. If antenatal diagnosis were to be confined to only four observations, measurement of hPL would be one of them.

Placental function tests in antenatal care

Table 8.1 Relative risk, predictive value and sensitivity for the more important factors observed in antenatal care (Grudzinskas et al. 1981). PET, pre-eclampsia; EH, essential hypertension; TP, true positive; FP, false positive; TN, true negative; FN, false negative.

Factor	Predictive value %	Sensitivity %	Relative risk (and P value)	TP/TP FN/FN	+	FP TN	+	Spontaneous labour %
White collar worker	6	10	0.6	17/273	:	155/1577		63
Non-smoker	8	54	0.6 (<0.001)	108/1428	:	93/682		59
hPL Groups 4 and 5	6	8	0.7	13/221	:	146/1663		56
Mild/moderate E.H. (diastolic BP 90–110 mmHg)	7	2	0.7	4/58	:	189/2006		36
Maternal age <20 years	8	8	0.8	17/213	:	186/1915		64
Threatened abortion	9	5	1.0	10/110	:	189/1997		63
Unskilled worker	9	37	1.0	64/684	:	108/1166		57
Mild/moderate PET (diastolic BP 90–110 mmHg)	9	11	1.0	22/284	:	171/1819		38
Professional occupation	9	13	1.0	23/244	:	149/1606		59
Non-white	10	9	1.1	18/178	:	185/1950		75
Skilled manual worker	10	33	1.2	57/543	:	115/1307		57
Previous perinatal death	11	9	1.3	8/74	:	78/973		52
Fetal biparietal diameter <10th centile[a]	12	13	1.5	13/105	:	88/1063		51
Maternal disease[b]	14	9	1.5	18/133	:	185/1988		51
1–15 cigarettes per day at booking	12	31	1.6 (<0.01)	49/398	:	108/1428		56
>15 cigarettes per day at booking	16	21	1.7 (<0.01)	41/250	:	157/1669		61
Raised maternal AFP	18	5	1.9	7/40	:	147/1606		66
Meconium staining of amniotic fluid in labour	17	19	2.0 (<0.001)	33/196	:	142/1726		56
Maternal age >34 years	20	12	2.2 (<0.001)	24/123	:	179/2005		54
Confirmed antepartum haemorrhage	22	7	2.4 (<0.01)	13/60	:	185/2040		57
Fetal heart rate abnormality (in first stage of labour)	19	23	2.4 (<0.001)	41/218	:	137/1724		40
hPL Groups 1 and 2 (<10th centile)	18	22	2.5 (<0.001)	35/194	:	124/1690		75
hPL Groups 1 (consistently <10th centile)	25	17	3.4 (<0.001)	27/106	:	132/1778		39
Severe PET and H.E. (diastolic BP >110 mmHg or proteinuria)	56	3	6.0 (<0.001)	5/9	:	194/2092		0

[a]Week 18–22 [b]Cardiac, renal, bowel, endocrine.

The evidence of Table 8.1, and that of many other studies, leaves no doubt that placental function tests give positive clinical information. The remaining question is whether this information is worth having. Will it make any difference to the outcome of pregnancy if the clinician knows that a patient has a low hPL? In the study described here low hPL was clearly associated with clinical action: an induction rate of 61%, which was only greatly exceeded by that in severe pre-eclampsia (100%). However, another high action group (62% induction rate) was mild hypertension, which was not associated with any increase in fetal risk. Clearly therefore, the fact that a test gave rise to a positive clinical response is no guide to the real value of the test.

There is only one study which has examined critically whether a placental function test is worth doing. Spellacy et al. (1975) examined 2733 subjects with clinical evidence of fetal risk. hPL levels were measured in all subjects, but the results reported to the clinician in only half. In the reported group the perinatal mortality was 3.4%, in the unreported group, 15%. This type of investigation would well merit repeating, although there would be considerable ethical problems about a test already well recognised as part of antenatal care. Nevertheless, it is remarkable that this is the only study of any parameter which has been examined in a randomised trial. No one, for example, has ever shown whether a knowledge of the patient's history or blood pressure makes any difference to fetal outcome. It is assumed that these are useful because they are related to outcome, but it has not been demonstrated that the knowledge will affect the outcome. Those who criticise the scientific approach to antenatal care as unproven should at least be aware that most traditional parameters are equally unproven, and that such arguments can readily be extended to show that most antenatal observations are unnecessary.

Interpretation of placental function tests

The interpretation of biochemical tests of placental function is, in truth, very simple and with few exceptions proceeds as follows. The measured level in an individual patient is compared with the normal range for that particular week of gestation. If the level is below normal limits it suggests, but does not guarantee, that the fetus is at risk; if the level is within normal limits it suggests, but again does not guarantee, that the fetus is not at risk. Exceptions to this generalisation are noted below under the headings of the specific complications.

Threatened abortion

Except for alphafetoprotein (where elevated levels are the unfavourable sign) concentrations of all fetoplacental products tend to be low in cases of threatened abortion in which the fetus is at risk. Levels can, therefore, be interpreted according to the simple rules given above. There are two main reservations. First, no biochemical test is particularly efficient prior to 6 weeks' gestation, and maximum diagnostic value is not achieved until 10 weeks or later, when the process leading to abortion may be far advanced. Second, a very accurate estimate of gestational age is needed because the levels of all fetoplacental products increase very rapidly up to 9 weeks and an error of only 1 week in dating can lead to substantial errors of interpretation. For the same reason serial estimations are of particular value in this situation: failure of levels to rise over a period of 1 week when normally they should more than double is a notably unfavourable sign.

Ectopic pregnancy

The only function of biochemical studies in ectopic gestation is to provide a simple qualitative test of the presence or absence of a pregnancy—a very useful procedure in cases of lower abdominal pain of uncertain aetiology (Seppälä et al. 1980).

Intrauterine growth retardation

Concentrations of fetoplacental products tend to be low in cases of intra-uterine growth retardation, and the best studies have consistently shown test sensitivities of the order of 25%–60%. In the third trimester it is unlikely that alternative diagnostic methods—manual examination and ultrasound—are any more efficient, though ultrasound offers the future promise of great accuracy and hence may replace other techniques.

There are two small exceptions to simple interpretations. Elevated alpha-fetoprotein levels in the second trimester are associated with reduced birth-weight in the third trimester. Elevated PP5 levels in the third trimester are characteristic of growth retardation with hypertension.

Hypertension and pre-eclampsia

Since placental function tests provide a general marker of fetal wellbeing, it is not surprising that the levels of fetoplacental products are often reduced in cases of hypertension and pre-eclampsia. But the important practical question is whether this information contributes to the overall management of the case. In other words, given that a diagnosis of pre-eclampsia has already been made, does it add anything to know whether the results of a biochemical test are normal or abnormal? There is, in fact, no well-documented answer to this simple question; most published studies simply address the difference in test levels between pre-eclamptic subjects and normals, rather than differences within the pre-eclamptic group itself. However, it is our general impression that the interpretation of test results is very similar to that in other clinical conditions, albeit with a rather higher incidence of abnormal findings. Thus, if a patient has diagnosed pre-eclampsia and hence an increased fetal risk, the finding of a low level of a placental product further increases this risk while a normal level would reduce it. Placental function tests, therefore, do have an important role in the management of such cases.

It should also be noted that evidence is accumulating for the existence of elevated levels of certain placental products in pre-eclampsia (e.g. PP5 and PAPP-A). The practical significance of this remains to be determined.

Diabetic mothers

Interpretation of placental function tests in diabetic mothers has been much confused by the failure to appreciate that elevated levels are to be expected. For this reason a result in the lower end of the normal range becomes an unfavourable sign. To add to the problems, current management of diabetes in pregnancy has become so efficient in metabolic terms that the pregnancy is effectively normal from the obstetric point of view. Thus, it is not surprising that some recent studies have shown normal levels of placental products in association with a normal outcome of pregnancy (Grudzinskas et al. 1981). In a well-run unit, therefore, interpretation of placental function tests in a diabetic pregnancy should probably be identical to that in a non-diabetic patient.

Rhesus isoimmunisation

Rhesus isoimmunisation is now a rare problem in obstetrics. Two applications of placental function tests have been suggested. First, elevated levels of placental proteins in the second trimester may predict the severity of the condition (see Chap. 6). Second, low or drastically falling levels may indicate fetal demise. There is no sound evidence that placental function tests in Rhesus isoimmunisation are useful in either context and much suggests that they may on occasion be misleading (Klopper and Stephenson 1966).

Intrauterine fetal death

Modern methods for detecting the fetal heartbeat are so sensitive and reliable that there is no place for placental function tests for detecting fetal death after the event. The key is the capacity of placental function tests to signal impending fetal death. This is not a question which lends itself to a general answer. The fetus may die in utero for many reasons; different ones will affect different placental function tests in different ways. In the end there are only two mechanisms of fetal death: something goes amiss with the fetus, it dies, the umbilical circulation stops, but the placenta, nourished from the maternal circulation, survives, at least in morphological terms. Or, the primary event may be placental, as when a placenta praevia is detached from the uterus wall. Often the two processes go hand in hand, although they usually start in the placenta. Placental proteins such as hPL are synthesised wholly in the trophoblast without input or control from the fetus. Placental pathology will affect them; fetal lesions will presumably not do so. In the case of steroids such as oestriol, the placenta cannot synthesise the compound without a supply of precursor from the fetus. In practice this distinction between fetus and placenta is blurred. Because oestriol has both fetal and placental elements in its genesis, serial assays of this steroid are marginally better than hPL measurements as a warning of impending fetal death, but there is little to choose between the two.

Acute fetal distress or neonatal asphyxia

It is a vexed question whether placental function tests will predict acute fetal distress or neonatal asphyxia and, if even they do, it is still difficult to ascertain the sensitivity, predictive value, etc. Rather than discussing this at length we will put forward two general conclusions: (1) in cases in which the fetal anoxia is due exclusively to mechanical events during labour (e.g. prolonged labour) or to prematurity, placental function tests will have no predictive value; (2) in cases in which the fetal anoxia is merely part of a long-term nutritional deprivation of the fetus (as evidenced, for example, by growth retardation) placental function tests will have predictive value. Failure to distinguish these two situations (which, in truth, is not easy) may explain much of the confusion in published studies. The final conclusion is that placental function tests will predict some but not all cases of acute fetal distress, the 'some' being difficult to define.

Prolonged pregnancy

There is little doubt that at and after term placental function deteriorates. Sometimes the process is rapid, sometimes slow. Almost always it is placental in origin. Placental function tests, particularly those associated with placental as opposed to fetal function, reflect rapid placental deterioration and are useful. In prolonged pregnancy, the obstetrician is often willing to accept trivial changes as a cause to induce labour. A single low value may legitimately tip the balance.

Maternal smoking

Maternal smoking is associated with a wide range of fetal risks, especially growth retardation, which can be predicted by placental function tests. The practical question is whether interpretation of results is any different between smokers and non-smokers, i.e. should a low value be taken more seriously in a smoker? This does not appear to be the case (Lee et al. 1980).

Premature labour

None of the well-known placental function tests will predict premature labour (though levels may vary with some of the associated complications such as pre-eclampsia). This is not surprising when one considers that such patients are to all intents and purposes normal until some unidentified event precipitates the onset of uterine contractions.

However, there is some evidence that high levels of PP5 and PAPP-A (see Chap. 7) are associated with premature labour. These findings require confirmation, but are of obvious importance if true.

Placental function tests as screening tests

Fetal risk represents a spectrum of different events (see Table 1.1). Antenatal observations are another spectrum and there is rarely, if ever, a 1:1 relationship between the two. Thus, an abnormal observation may or may not be associated with fetal risk, and fetal risk may or may not be associated with an abnormal observation. This being the case, there is no reason why any parameter should have unique diagnostic value, or to suggest that if one parameter is normal all others will also be normal. Antenatal care consists of the accumulation of a series of independent observations—a multi-parameter screening process.

Some antenatal observations are used as routine screening tests (e.g. blood pressure, urine testing). Others, for no very obvious reason, are not, despite the fact that they may yield information of equivalent value; the placental function tests are one of these. We have argued that placental function tests should be used on a routine screening basis, because there is good evidence that they help to isolate a high-risk category and will occasionally identify cases not found by another means. In our view there is a good case to be made for doing at least a single test in every pregnancy. Many of the physiological adaptations of pregnancy reach their peak at 36 weeks. This is the optimal time to carry out placental function tests.

Choice of test

Nothing has generated more disagreement, not to say acrimony, than the question of 'which test?'. The fact that this argument has continued for two decades and is only fuelled by the introduction of new parameters suggests to us a simple conclusion: that subject to a few minor qualifications, *all tests are the same*. It remains only to state the qualifications, and to give some final recommendations to the individual clinician, who may be confused by the plethora of possibilities.

Choice of test

First trimester

The low levels of most fetoplacental products in early pregnancy suggest, a priori, that only materials presenting readily measurable concentrations at this time are likely to be of clinical value. This reduces the choice to five: hPL, hCG, SP1, oestrogens and progesterone. hPL assays have proved most useful in discriminating between inevitable abortion and a viable pregnancy; hCG assays have not lived up to their early promise in the management of abortion, but may now have a place in the diagnosis of very early abortion—implantation failure; SP1 is also measurable in very early pregnancy and when more is known about it, may prove to be valuable; progesterone, in spite of being quantitatively the main steroid of pregnancy, is too variable to give much information of value in pregnancy. Somewhat surprisingly, oestriol assays appear to be useful in women with a history of recurrent abortion, where they may give the earliest indication of impending disaster (Klopper and Macnaughton 1965).

Second trimester

By 12 weeks of pregnancy all fetoplacental products are easily measured by standard procedures and the 'all tests are identical' rule can probably be applied. However, only two tests have been sufficiently well documented to provide the basis for a recommendation: hPL and alphafetoprotein. Details of the application of these can be found in Chap. 6. The use of AFP in screening for neural tube defects is outside the scope of this book.

Third trimester

The third trimester is the high point of the argument. At one time or another, every test in this book has been advocated as a parameter of fetoplacental function in the last 12 weeks of gestation. Based on the twin criteria of availability and documentation, only two tests can be recommended: hPL and oestriol. All others can be dismissed on the grounds which have already been dealt with in individual chapters. However, the dismissal is not final: at a research level some of the new placental proteins—SP1, PAPP-A and PP5—have great promise; but this is for the future, not today.

In our view, there is little to choose between hPL and oestrogens in clinical terms. If a unit is conducting an hPL assay there is no obvious reason to switch to oestrogens, or vice versa. This presupposes that the technology used is precise, inexpensive and rapid. If a unit is not conducting such tests, but wishes to do so, then the choice between hPL and oestrogens is finely balanced, and the decision could be based on any one of a selection of ancillary criteria: laboratory preference, costs, etc. Better funded groups might choose to do both, though it could be argued that two estimates by one test is as good as one estimate by each of two tests.

References

Gordon YB, Lewis JD, Pendlebury DJ, Leighton M, Gold J (1978) Is measurement of placental function and maternal weight worthwhile? Lancet i: 1001

Grudzinskas JG, Gordon YB, Wadsworth J, Menabawey M, Chard T (1981) Is placental function testing worthwhile? An update on placental lactogen. Aust NZ J Obstet Gynaecol 21: 103

Klopper A, Macnaughton M (1965) Hormones in recurrent abortion. J Obstet Gynaecol Br Commonwealth 72: 1022

Klopper A, Stephenson R (1966) The excretion of oestriol and of pregnanediol in pregnancies complicated by Rh immunization. J Obstet Gynaecol Br Commonwealth 73: 282–289

Lee JN, Grudzinskas JG, Chard T (1980) Circulating placental lactogen (hPL) levels in relation to smoking during pregnancy. J Obstet Gynaecol 1: 87

Seppälä M, Tontti K, Ranta T, Stenman U-H, Chard T (1980) Use of a rapid hCG-beta-subunit radioimmunoassay in acute gynaecological emergencies. Lancet i: 165

Spellacy WN, Buhi WC, Birk SA (1975) The effectiveness of human placental lactogen as an adjunct in decreasing perinatal death. Am J Obstet Gynecol 121: 835

Subject Index

Abortion 86
    hCG levels 61-62
    hPL levels 63
    oestriol levels 50-51
    progesterone levels 50-51
    SP1 levels 73–74
Accuracy of assay 13
Amniotic fluid 8, 6
Aromatase 42, 45

Basement membrane 5–7, 15

Centiles 25
Chi-square test 27–28
Choice of test 90–91
Cholesterol 39, 42
Chorionic gonadotrophin (hCG) 46
    chemistry and synthesis 56–57
    clinical applications 60–63
    control 58–59
    functions 58
    measurement 59–60
    metabolism 57
    variability 60
Control mechanisms of placental products 11–12
Controlled studies 31, 67, 86
Cystine aminopeptidase 34–36

Dehydroepiandrosterone sulphate 11–12, 37, 42–43, 53
Diabetes 15, 88
    hPL levels 65
    oestriol levels 52
    SP1 levels 75
Distribution of placental products 7–8
Dynamic tests 53

Ectopic pregnancy 87
    hCG levels 62
Epioestriol 47

False negatives 26–27
False positives 26–27
Fetal capillaries 5–7, 14
Fetal death *see* Intrauterine death
Fetal distress
    hPL levels 66–67, 84–86
'Fetoplacental unit' 10, 42–43
Functions of placental products 10

Gaussian distribution 24–25

Half-life of placental products 8–9
Heat-stable alkaline phosphatase 34–36
Hydroxysteroid dehydrogenase 34, 37, 42

Intervillous space 5–7, 11, 16
Intrauterine death 89
    hPL levels 66
    oestriol levels 53
Intrauterine growth retardation 20–21, 87
    hPL levels 64
    oestriol levels 52–53
    PAPP-A levels 79
    PP5 levels 76–77
    SP1 levels 74–75

Kober reaction 39, 46

Maternal blood vessels 16

Subject Index

Measurement of placental products 12–14
Median 25
Metabolism of placental products 8–9
Multiples of median 25–26

Non-parametric distribution 25–26
Normal (definition of) 18–19
Normal ranges 18–19
    hPL 60–61
    oestriol 49–51
    PAPP-A 79
    PP5 77
    SP1 73

Oestetrol 53
Oestradiol 53
Oestriol 40–53
    clinical applications 50–53
    conjugation 43–44
    control 45–46
    function 44–45
    measurement 46–47
    metabolism 43–44
    variability 48–49

Perinatal mortality 1–3, 22, 31
Placental abruption 77
Placental lactogen
    chemistry and synthesis 56–57
    clinical applications 63–67, 83–87
    control 59
    functions 58
    measurement 59–60
    metabolism 57
    variability 60
Placental protein 5 (PP5)
    biology 76
    chemistry 76
    clinical applications 76–77
Placental transfer 6
Precision of assay 13
Predictive value 26–27
Pre-eclampsia 16, 20, 87–88
    hPL levels 64–65
    oestriol levels 52
    PAPP-A levels 79–80
    SP1 levels 75

Pregnancy-associated plasma protein A
(PAPP-A) 78–80
    clinical applications 79–80
    physiology 78–79
Pregnancy specific β_1 glycoprotein see
Schwangerschaftsprotein 1
Pregnanediol 53–54
Pregnenolone 40
Premature labour 77, 90
Progesterone 50–51, 53–54
Prolonged pregnancy 89
    hPL levels 67
Prospective surveys 30, 67

Radioimmunoassay 47
Relative risk ratio 29, 67
Rhesus isoimmunisation 15, 88
    hPL levels 65
    oestriol levels 53

Schwangerschaftsprotein 1 (SP1) 71–76
    chemistry 71
    clinical applications 73–76
    synthesis 71–72
    variability 72
Screening tests 67–68, 83–87, 90
Sensitivity of assay 12–13
Sensitivity of tests 27–28
Serial determinations 31–33
Smoking 67, 89
SP1 see Schwangerschaftsprotein 1
Specificity of assay 13
Sulphatase deficiency 10, 37
Synthesis of placental products 5–7

Trophoblast 5–7, 11–12, 15–16
True negatives 26–27
True positives 26–27

Urinary excretion 9
    choice of test 47–48

Variation of placental products 8–9, 29, 31–33
    hPL 60
    oestriol 48–49

by the same authors:

Placental Proteins

Editors: A.I.Klopper, T.Chard
1979. 65 figures, 36 tables. X, 171 pages
ISBN 3-540-09406-7

Contents: The Specific Proteins of the Human Placenta − Some New Hypotheses. − The Measurement of Trophoblastic Proteins as a Test of Placental Function. − Potential Antifertility Vaccines Using Antigens of hCG. − The Use of Antibody Affinity Chromatography and Other Methods in the Study of Pregnancy-Associated Proteins. − Isolation and Characterization of Placental Proteins with Special Reference to Pregnancy-Specific β_1 Glycoprotein (PSβG). − Practical and Theoretical Considerations in the Measurements of Pregnancy-Specific β_1 Glycoprotein. − Trophoblast-Specific β_1 Glycoproteins as an Indicator of Pregnancy and Neoplasia − A Review of Recent Clinical Studies.

This volume is the third to flow from the triennial conferences on the Endocrinology of Pregnancy held in Aberdeen. It is not, however, simply the proceedings of the meeting and does not, indeed, contain any discussion. It contains the substance of the eleven main lectures given by the distinguished research workers from all over the world who where invited to present their findings. The book consists, therefore, of a series of essays about various aspects of placental proteins. It is not a comprehensive review of all the pregnancy-associated proteins, but considers only pregnancy-specific proteins which do not occur in non-pregnant subjects. It concentrates largely upon three or four new proteins of trophoblastic origin whoch have been isolated in the last few years. Although their clinical significance is by no means clear, it is accepted that these proteins appear in increasing concentration in the maternal circulation during pregnancy. The purpose of this book is to explore the physiology of the new placental proteins, to document the results which have so far been obtained by their measurement in the blood of pregnant women, and to set forth data and speculation about the clinical application of such measurements.

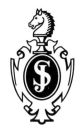

Springer-Verlag
Berlin
Heidelberg
NewYork

of related interest:

Functional Morphologic Changes in Female Sex Organs Induced by Exogenous Hormones
Editor: G. Dallenbach-Hellweg
1980. 139 figures, 42 tables.
XV, 234 pages
ISBN 3-540-09885-2

A. E. Schindler
Hormones in Human Amniotic Fluid
1982. 23 figures, 133 tables.
XII, 158 pages
(Monographs on Endocrinology, Volume 21)
ISBN 3-540-10810-6

J. H. Clark, E. J. Peck, Jr.
Female Sex Steroids
Receptors and Function
1979. 116 figures, 18 tables.
XII, 245 pages
(Monographs an Endocrinology, Volume 14)
ISBN 3-540-09375-3

P. J. Keller
Hormonal Disorder in Gynecology
Translated from the German by T. C. Telger
1981. 89 figures, 9 tables. IX, 113 pages
ISBN 3-540-10341-4

Pathology of the Female Genital Tract
Editor: A. Blaustein
2nd edition 1982. 1249 figures (39 in full color). XIX, 939 pages
ISBN 3-540-90574-X

G. Dallenbach-Hellweg
Histopathology of the Endometrium
English Translation by F. D. Dallenbach
3rd revised and updated edition.
1981. 147 figures, 2 colored plates.
VI, 359 pages
ISBN 3-540-10658-8

H. Elias
Human Embryology: Normal and Pathologic
With contributions by J. E. Pauly, C. B. Severn
1982. 450 figures. Approx. 680 pages
ISBN 3-540-06229-7

Cervical Cancer
Editor: G. Dallenbach-Hellweg
1981. 115 figures. VIII, 259 pages
(Current Topics in Pathology, Volume 70)
ISBN 3-540-10941-2

H. Ludwig, H. Metzger
The Human Female Reproductive Tract
A Scanning Electron Microscopic Atlas
1976. 546 micrographs. XI, 247 pages
ISBN 3-540-07675-1

Chronic Pelvic Pain in Women
Editor: M. Renaer
1981. 22 figures, 10 tables.
XIII, 197 pages
ISBN 3-540-10608-1

Springer-Verlag
Berlin
Heidelberg
New York

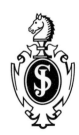